ISOMETRIC POWER PULSE

Method

ISOMETRIC POWER PULSE

Method

The Best Isometric system that build muscle, increase strength, burn fat and sculpt the best body without the use of weights!

BECOME RIPPED!

The Isometric Power Pulse Method was written to help you get closer to your physical potential when it comes to real muscle sculpting strengthening exercises. The exercises and routines in this book are quite demanding, so consult your physician and have a physical exam taken prior to the start of this exercise program. Proceed with the suggested exercises and information at your own risk. The Publishers and author shall not be liable or responsible for any loss, injury, or damage allegedly arising from the information or suggestions in this book.

Isometric Power Pulse Method
muscle-building Course

By

Birch Tree Publishing
Published by Birch Tree Publishing

Birch Tree Publishing

Dedication

For everyone that want to enhance their body, this book is for **YOU!**

Contents

Introduction: DEVELOP A POWERFUL RIPPED BODY   **PG 7**

Chapter 1: ISOMETRIC POWER PULSES   **PG 12**

Chapter 2: SCULPT A RIPPED CHEST   **PG 18**

Chapter 3: DEVELOP RIPPED SHOULDERS   **PG 21**

Chapter 4: DEVELOP A POWERFUL V-TAPER   **PG 26**

Chapter 5: DEVELOP POWERFUL NECK MUSCLES   **PG 33**

Chapter 6: BUILD BASEBALL SHAPED BICEPS   **PG 39**

Chapter 7: DEVELOP POWERFUL TRICEPS   **PG 45**

Chapter 8: DEVELOP RIPPED FOREARMS   **PG 50**

Chapter 9: LEGS/LOWER BACK HAMSTRINGS   **PG 53**

Chapter 10: DEVELOP SHAPELY CALVES   **PG 60**

Chapter 11: DEVELOP RIPPED ABS   **PG 63**

Chapter 12: ULTIMATE POWER PULSE METHOD   **PG 69**

Chapter 13: ULTIMATE FAT-LOSS POWER MAX PROGRAM   **PG 80**

Chapter 14: ENHANCING MUSCLE FIBER ACTIVATION   **PG 88**

Chapter 15: THE ISOMETRIC FAT-LOSS PLAN   **PG 100**

Chapter 16: THE ISOMETRIC POWER 10 PROGRAM   **PG 122**

Chapter 17: Isometric Power PULSE X40 PROGRAM   **PG 134**

GET ISOMETRIC RIPPED

And now, the worlds fastest muscle-building method

Introduction by Marlon Birch

The Isometric Power Pulse Method increases lean muscle with powerful Isometric routines that deliver results. You will be amazed at how quickly your muscle size will increase, right in the comfort of your own home. You will see and feel your muscles getting leaner while gaining strength to your arms, neck and lower back muscles.

My program will build lean muscle much faster with effective isometric training. The Isometric Power Pulse Method are quick 20 minute power-packed routines that increase muscle and strength, right before your very eyes. You will realise how quickly your body will change, in fact in just minutes per day. I've been helping hundreds of men and women just like you to get in shape since 1995, and I've learned what it takes to get the body of your dreams in the shortest time possible.

This book introduces The Ultimate Isometric Power Pulse Workouts these programs will get you in the best shape **FASTER** than you thought possible. With the power of our system and the muscle-building benefits of powerful Isometric holds. Combining a phase approach with Isometric Pulses force the muscles to contract harder and over come neuromuscular system failure.

My Isometric system extend and enhance overload on the muscles, and you will see muscle popping up almost overnight. While getting more muscular and leaner than ever before. It's an eye-opening program that can help you pack on muscle and strength fast. The Isometric Power Pulse Method is exactly what you need to focus on attaining that ripped, lean and powerful build.

I remember back in the day Charles Atlas was the only fitness authority everyone wanted to be and look like. I followed in his footsteps along with millions of young men and women. Charles Atlas was getting the world in shape with a simple protocol that included self resistance and calisthenics along with a great attitude!

I am not Charles Atlas, but my Isometric Power Pulse Method will work for you because it's based on sound fundamental basics. It is by far the safest method for developing muscles, gaining strength and increasing power with Isometric exercises safely. I remember as a teenager, my uncle tensed his forearm muscles in a way that seemed surreal to me.

At first, all I saw were veins and ripped cords of muscle. He said grab my arm and squeeze it. I then felt the layers of muscle tense from inner to outer, like an inflated balloon being blown up. My uncle's forearm muscles were fully engaged; it felt like his forearm had turned to granite from what I remember. Normally, when you squeeze someones' arm, even when they are tense, there is some softness to the outer layers of tissue.

My Uncle explained that he had developed a high level of control over his muscles throughout the years. He turned to me and said tense, so I did, and he told me that when most people tense up, they use only a fraction of their muscle fibers. My Uncle said that people's inability to control more of their muscle fibers limited their functionality and strength. He stated to develop true strength one need to master the tension at will inside the muscle itself.

Months later I realised the greater the force generation and control, the greater muscle gains you will receive. This Isometric book will teach you how to control your muscles, for we have so much more control than we realise.. This form of training will build you from the inside out.

Meaning, you will control not only your muscles, but your emotions as well. Simple issues will not bother you any more. The more you practice, the more control you will gain in every aspect of your life. That is the foundation of the program. The key is to incorporate the principles of Isometric Power into your daily routine. You will gain greater control over your life and learn how to let things go that you really need to. This element took awhile for me to develop, but when you do, it is the key to self mastery.

I do not base this on controlling everything in your life. It is about controlling your reaction to various situations you face on a day-to-day basis, so you can procure and experience greater fulfillment and joy in your life. Consistent effort along with a positive mental attitude–coupled with this well-thought-out muscle-building-exercise plan, is all you need to acquire your goal - even after your first workout! That's why this routine book was put together.

Yours In Strength and Power
Marlon Birch

LET'S BEGIN

LET'S BEGIN

If you are reading this book, you already appreciate the importance of exercising for health, strength and well being. The Isometric Power Pulse Program will turn you into a powerful well built man. Let's face it, being a great success at exercising means constant practice to transform yourself to become the best you can be.

Of course, when it comes to training-like most everything else in life-sometimes circumstances seem to get in the way from allowing you to exercise. Now, thanks to Power Pulse, you will always get a great workout-no matter where you are.

Isometric strength training with Isometric Power Pulses enhances:

1) Isometric strength training stimulates muscles to burn more calories than anything else. After your workout your metabolism is triggered for 40 hours after the session.
2) Your body will take on a different shape, and your clothes will fit far better.
3) Your flexibility will increase and resistance training will keep you young.
4) Your bones will become stronger. We lose bone mass as we get older, but resistance strength training increases bone density and add greater strength.
5) A stronger and healthy heart with enhanced blood flow.
6) Stress levels will be reduced due to exercise.
7) Resistance strength training also creates better sleeping patterns.
8) "No need to get depressed". Regular resistance training will ward off symptoms of depression.
9) Mental sharpness will be developed. This takes place due resistance training decreasing blood levels of homocysteine, the protein that's linked to developing Alzheimer's and dementia. Plus, resistance training enhances cognitive function. Workouts will improve memory and you will have longer attention spans.
10) Develop lazar-like focus.

The Isometric method that will create

a

RIPPED

Isometric Body

Chapter 1:
ISOMETRIC POWER PULSES

How Power Pulses increase strength, help you lose bodyfat and develop powerful muscles.

Create the body of your dreams NOW!

01 ISOMETRIC POWER PULSES

The Isometric Power Pulse Method will turn your body into an efficient muscle-sculpting-fat-burning machine. Everyone is trying to improve their physique to get firmer, stronger, with lower bodyfat levels. However, this can be quite a challenging job for most, when it comes to the body adapting to new stress, the more irritation it receives the more the body resists. The only reason Mother Nature will back down is if those muscles are absolutely necessary for everyday use and survival. The biggest road-block is your nervous system and adaptation.

Within this book there are specific phases to increase and coax muscle growth and strength gains for every bodypart, but the nervous system comes into play once your muscles hit muscular failure. This leaves loads of muscle fibers that do not get the stimulation that they need to promote muscle growth.

This is where the Isometric Power Pulse Method comes into play to boast those endurance fibers into firing rapidly, that will allow the trainee to ramp up the stress placed on the muscles for added progress to follow. I've put together the best programs that stimulate the strongest-muscle-building-signal to ensure effective stimulation of the muscles to coax greater muscle fiber recruitment and growth on every rep.

However, in my quest to educate trainees all over the world they can do set after set, but may never quite hit that anabolic drive that they need to progress. Using the best mass-building exercises is only part of the anabolic solution. Over the years I've heard trainees ask before they get onboard with me, Marlon I have been doing set after set of these exercises with little improvement for my efforts. This is where I came in and taught them the patterns of irritating the muscle fibers to force recruitment of the motor units to fire efficiently.

In a regular set, low threshold units are recruited first (**type I slow-twitchers**, then the fast twitchers (**type II fibers**) at the last bit of the exercise set. However, most times those fibers are never really stimulated for growth because the nervous system shuts down long before even touching those important (get big fibers) for muscle growth to take place.

01 ISOMETRIC POWER PULSES

This is where the Isometric Power Pulse muscle-building methods comes in, this coax the nervous system to take a back seat long enough to make that set 100 times more effective in getting at those hard to reach endurance fast twitchers to promote additional muscle-building-growth effect with Isometrics.

So the Isometric Power Pulse Method extends time under load on those endurance fast twitchers *in the strongest muscle-stimulating position of the movement* to increase fiber overload by coaxing hormonal release for a growth increase.
What is the Isometric Power Pulses Method? Basically, it is science meeting isometrics at the best Isometric system for promoting **REAL** muscle-growth.
The Isometric Power Pulse Method
In my quest to learn more about isometrics I developed a system that was applied at the age of 15 years old at the middle section of the exercise stroke on my curls this was in 1989. I realised that it worked well on a lot of the exercises. Some of my methods created more force generation than others while other holds significantly increased more effective muscle growth and leanness from increasing fiber overload.

At a very young age I realised that a trainee can make significant progress performing the isometric exercises a certain way, combined with extended stress methods tagged on for each exercise. This activated extreme fiber recruitment, which prolonged each set at a point where the target muscle is being stimulated with the best muscle-building impulse to contract those muscles at its maximum.

By using Power Pulse Isometric contractions on each muscle group the trainee will make significant gains in ripped, enhanced new muscle and strength rapidly. Your muscles will be filled with new powerful pumps from the very first exercise, by applying the Isometric Power Method to every exercise at the growth producing power point for coaxing muscle stimulation and growth.

My method of performing the Power Pulse protocol force more endurance fast-twitch fiber recruitment patterns. It's a better way of prolonging load time on the muscles and preventing nervous system failure it's the nervous system that shuts down, not the muscles being targeted.

01 ISOMETRIC POWER PULSES

The Power Pulses coax the nervous system to keep firing those endurance fast twitchers that contain the most growth potential *at the critical point at contracting those muscles* which increases the hormonal stimuli far greater than regular isometrics.

One method is Power Pulses. This will be explained later......However, by performing power pulses in a phase approach this increases fiber output and stresses the fibers to fire rapidly. This form of training force as many fibers to be stimulated, which develop as many muscle fibers as possible for max muscle size and strength. You will gain rapid fiber stimulation in developing all the fiber types to the max due to extended fiber overload with **(Time Under Load Expansion)!**

Let me just say that stopping the isometric contraction too short will do nothing for increasing fiber overload and growth production. So a 7-10 second Isometric contraction will never be recommended in my routines and programs, because low second holds do nothing for muscle growth. It will stimulate strength but, the only fiber types are stimulated are the power fibers, so low second isometrics will not hit the get big triggers to increase and coax muscle size.

The trainee will build strength more than anything and will develop sore tendons and ligaments. To build the muscle, the trainee need to stimulate the muscle fully by building all fiber types. There are so many types of fast, slow, medium and endurance twitch fibers, so the trainee must focus on developing all of them for complete development. This book will get the job done.

My Experience

Alot of you know my story but let me share with you guys on how my Isometric incarnation originated. In my experience I realised that low isometric holds became (old) fast! Plus, most times with my early experiments with training in the late 80s and early 90s, a lot of my fibers were unstimulated for muscle growth to be established. After a while adaptation takes place and the muscles stop responding for change to occur to promote muscle growth.

01 ISOMETRIC POWER PULSES

So I started performing isometric holds at various angles and hold times with my curls at the right spot in the range of motion this combination took a regular isometric exercise and forced more muscle-stimulation, coaxed more fibers and increased the time under load on the muscles within that contraction.

With my various isometric methods, I got maximum muscle-building stimulation at the power spot or precise position that stimulates the Greatest muscle-building signal of any isometric move for fiber activation in any one set. There was a serious increase in muscle growth, leanness and strength gains, with only a handful of sets.

I couldn't believe, with only 2 weeks of this method of training, I looked wider, got more vascular and was bigger than ever. My exercises became more intense, and the pump was out of this world. This was with power packed isometrics only. This got me motivated and my intensity was high with my isometric experiments. I must say that I was flawed by the results!

Isometric Power Pulses: How I Intensified my sets

Step 1: Lets look at a regular bicep curl, place the arm at 90 degrees and perform 1 second Isometric contractions in a piston pumping action. Contract release, contract release, and so on. At the (mid-point) this is where the strongest stimulation for that muscle while performing these Mini-Isometric-Power-Reps.

Isometric Power Pulses For Everyone

Even rank beginners can use the Power Pulse stress method workouts to break into a muscle-building and strengthening program, but you don't want to start out too hard, or you'll do too much tendon damage. Use a light to medium resistance (tension). Always remember, **Stimulate** the muscles, do not **annihilate** them!

Power Pulses increase fiber overload throughout the full range of muscle flexion. This form of training teaches the muscle how to contract at its optimum for increased development by procuring the pump with continuous mini-Isometric contractions. By combining Isometric Pulses to the contracted-position exercises, this supercharge the effectiveness of the movements by teaching the muscles to contract at its maximum.

01 ISOMETRIC POWER PULSES

Isometrics, combined with an Isolation exercise, program the targeted muscle to contract and activate more fibers per contraction. Stretch contracted exercises provide unique stress to the muscle fibers being trained, which stimulates strength gains. This increases Growth hormone production, setting up a greater anabolic environment for muscle growth to take place.

Later on within these pages you will see the Power Pulse Method tagged onto stretch-and contracted-position exercises. The most important part of the stroke for each exercise are the Isolation and (muscle-teamwork exercises).

My Isometric Power Pulse Program

Once the Isometric Pulses are introduced, your muscle size sky will skyrocket. The volume of exercises and sets will be cut in half to compensate for the intensity caused by the stress method, so that means shorter 15-20 minute effective workouts. As most readers know, I've been doing Isometric exercises for over 30 years.

So when it comes to results and effective training programs, which will make you work each muscle from one or two specific positions to ensure optimum-muscle-activation. The Isometric Power-Phases are effective.

However, I've made it even better and faster based on my experimentation and research. It's the perfect solution to a condensed program, making it even more efficient at increasing lean, ripped to the bone muscles. Practice and consistency is the name of the game here for self mastery.

What is Isometrics? Isometrics are exercises where your joints do not move. Normally with isotonic exercises, you move your joints through a full or partial range of motion. Lets look at a regular curl for example. You start off with the arm extended, then you slowly pull your arm upwards, then reverse the action. With an isometric exercise, you stay in a fixed position.

Chapter 2:

CHEST

SCULPT A RIPPED CHEST

SCULPT A RIPPED CHEST

02 SCULPT A RIPPED CHEST

The chest muscles allow you to push or move the arm forward or across the body. These muscles are activated in any throwing or pushing motion. Aesthetically, building a powerful chest is a sign of power in men.

However the chest muscles are not used on a daily basis, so most times they are under developed. So despite,the simplicity of how these muscles contract, they can be trained in a number of various angles of push and pull, each offer its own special muscle enhancing properties.

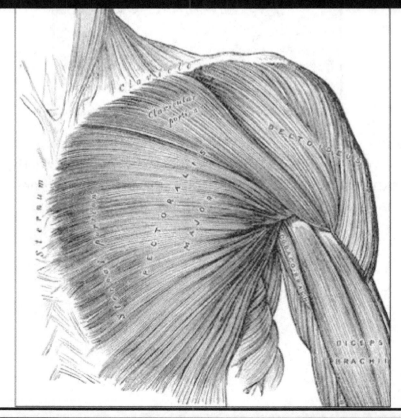

CHEST EXERCISES

02 SCULPT A RIPPED CHEST

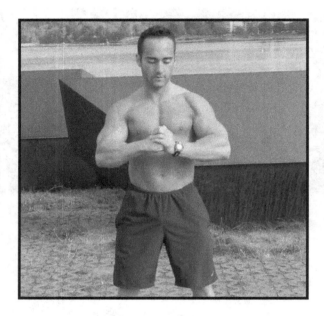

ISOMETRIC CHEST PRESS

This is an awesome building and shaping movement. Works the entire chest as well as the shoulders and triceps musculature. Press Isometrically right palm against the left and hold for desired seconds.

Chapter 3:

SHOULDERS
DEVELOP RIPPED SHOULDERS

DEVELOP RIPPED SHOULDERS

03 DEVELOP RIPPED SHOULDERS

The shoulder muscles are divided into three heads and are quite unique and move the arm in all directions. The front muscle raises the arm for ward, the side muscles made up of variable number of muscle bundles, and raises the arm out to the sides. The rear or posterior muscle, is designed to pull the arm backwards. Isometric forward raises are isolation exercise, which recruits the front and side heads of the shoulders that tie in well with stimulating the upper and mid-back muscles as well giving the entire girdle complete development.

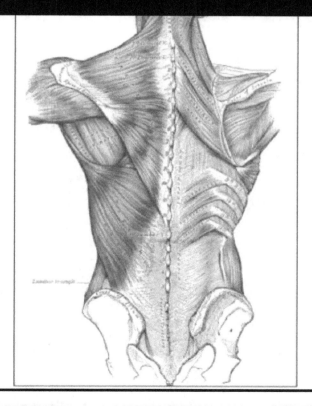

SHOULDER EXERCISES

03 DEVELOP RIPPED SHOULDERS

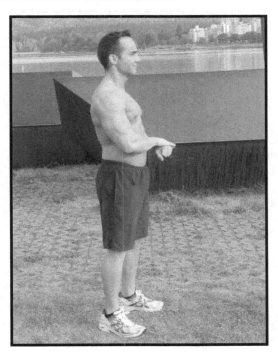

ISOMETRIC FORWARD RAISES

Grasp the right hand with the left in front of the body as shown. Isometrically raise the arm forward against the resistance of the other hand. Switch arms and continue. This works the front and side shoulder muscles.

SHOULDER EXERCISES

03 DEVELOP RIPPED SHOULDERS

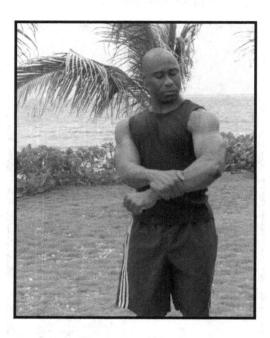

ISOMETRIC LATERAL RAISES

Grasp the left arm that is across the body as in the picture. Now raise the arm outwards towards the side contracted position, Isometrically resisting with the right arm.

SHOULDER EXERCISES

03 DEVELOP RIPPED SHOULDERS

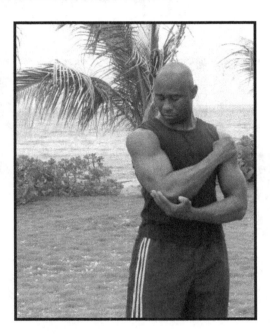

ACROSS THE BODY PULLS

Bring the right elbow across the body and grasp the left elbow with a firm grip. Isometrically press the right arm downwards while resisting with the left hand. This exercise adds strength and development to the rear shoulder muscles and upper back.

Chapter 4:

UPPER BACK
DEVELOP A POWERFUL V-TAPER

DEVELOP A POWERFUL V-TAPER

04 DEVELOP A POWERFUL V-TAPER

The entire back is made up of numerous muscles overlapping each other. Most trainees find the back quite difficult to fully develop. The reason? As the saying goes, out of sight, out of mind. We cannot directly see the back muscles, plus we cannot see it flex like we would see the biceps.

We make training the entire back musculature much easier making developing the back obviously simple once you know what you are doing, you can bring these muscles up to speed. We are looking at the large Latissimus that covers the majority of the back. The trapezius is broken up into two sections.

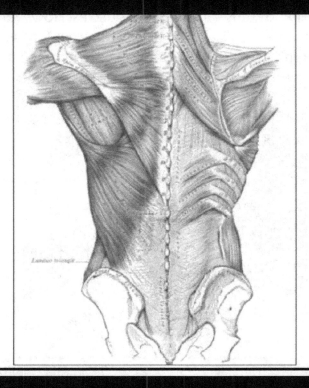

UPPER BACK EXERCISES

04 DEVELOP A POWERFUL V-TAPER

DO NOT NEGLECT THE MID AND LOWER TRAPS

Theres the upper traps and mid-back muscles. Plus we have the teres major, which is strongly stimulated as well, which makes Isometrics the ideal exercise. The infraspinatus muscle is like a half circle on each side of the upper back and is a very important rotator cuff muscle.

This muscle stabilize the shoulder and prevent dislocations. Even though this muscle is at the back, most traditional exercises do not fully target these muscles. However with our plans there are exercises that target this area for full development.

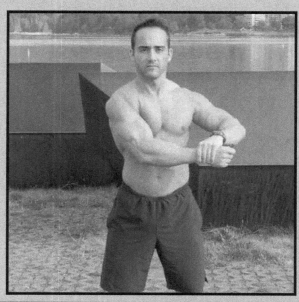

UPPER BACK EXERCISES

04 DEVELOP A POWERFUL V-TAPER

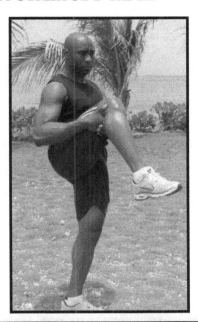

ISOMETRIC THIGH ROWS

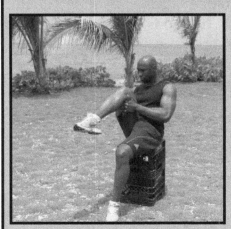

Interlock the fingers behind the knee as shown with right leg. With both arms pull the thigh upwards towards the chest while resisting with the leg. If balance is an issue perform the exercise seated.

UPPER BACK EXERCISES

04 DEVELOP A POWERFUL V-TAPER

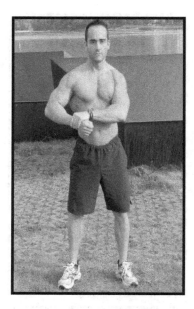

ISOMETRIC ROWS

Maintain position, grasp the wrist with the left hand. Isometrically pull the hand toward the right against the resistance supplied by the left hand. Repeat the movement then switch arms. This adds thickens to the mid back and lats, along with the rear part of the shoulders.

UPPER BACK EXERCISES

04 DEVELOP A POWERFUL V-TAPER

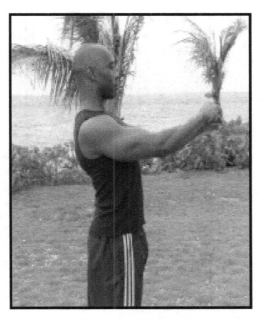

ISOMETRIC STIFF ARM PULLDOWNS

Grasp the left hand with the right as in the picture. Isometrically push the arm downwards while resisting with the bottom arm. Works the upper-back.

UPPER BACK EXERCISES

04 DEVELOP A POWERFUL V-TAPER

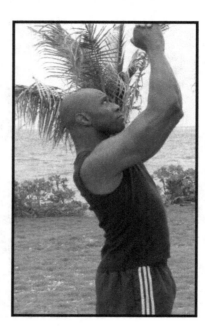

ISOMETRIC PULLDOWNS

With the arms over-head place your left hand on top of the right fist as shown. Isometrically pull down with the left hand resisting with the right, once finished switch arms.

Chapter 5:

TRAPS/NECK
DEVELOP POWERFUL NECK MUSCLES

DEVELOP POWERFUL TRAPS

05 DEVELOP POWERFUL TRAPS/MID-BACK

The trapezuis muscles are in three parts: The upper traps, this lifts the shoulder girdle, the (bottom-traps, which works in opposition to the upper traps. Lowers the shoulders. The middle traps (mid-back) which along with the rhomboids that partially covers, bring the shoulder blades together.

With isometrics exercises the upper traps will look impressive in clothes and will add a complete look to your upper body. Making it more balanced. Our Isometric method of exercise will avoid imbalances between the upper and mid-trap muscles. Complete development takes place due to an efficient training program.

A lot of our various exercises stimulate various sections of the muscles. Which prevents an imbalance of the upper traps becoming far too developed than the mid-back and lower-traps muscles. It's important to know that the lower traps stabilize and protect the shoulder girdle.

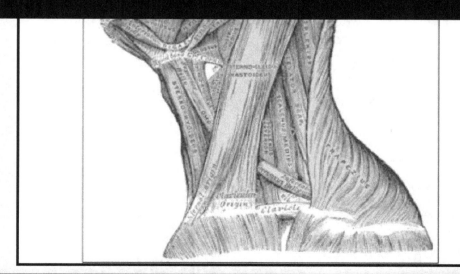

TRAPEZUIS EXERCISES

05 DEVELOP POWERFUL TRAPS/MID-BACK

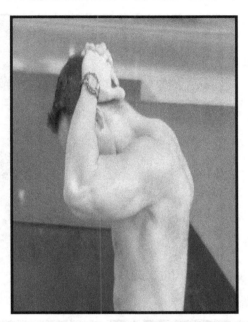

REAR NECK PRESS

Place your hands behind your head and tuck the chin on the upper chest as shown. Now Isometrically press the head against the hand while resisting with your hands.
Use a light tension at the beginning and increase the tension to medium as you get stronger and more conditioned.

TRAPEZUIS EXERCISES

05 DEVELOP POWERFUL TRAPS/MID-BACK

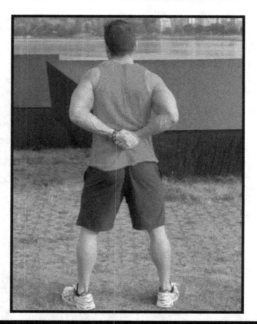

ISOMETRIC REVERSE UPRIGHT ROW

Place your arm behind your back as shown. Hold onto the wrist with the other hand lean forward a-little and Isometrically pull the right arm upwards while resisting with the right hand. This works the mid-back, upper traps and rear delts.

TRAPEZUIS EXERCISES

05 DEVELOP POWERFUL TRAPS/MID-BACK

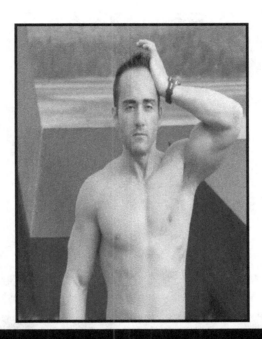

ISOMETRIC SIDE NECK PRESS

As shown above, place your hands on your head and push the head against the hand. Hold the position Isometrically for the desired seconds. This exercise stimulates the side muscles of the neck.

TRAPEZUIS EXERCISES

05 DEVELOP POWERFUL TRAPS/MID-BACK

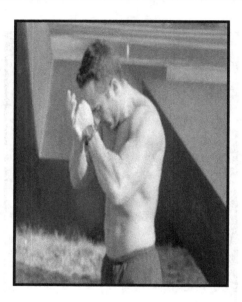

ISOMETRIC FRONT NECK PRESS

With your head tilted forward place your hand on your forehead. Now push your head forward and resist the movement Isometrically with light tension. Always use a light tension to the neck.

As your strength increases use a little more force but not too much tension. **Breathe Normal.**

Chapter 6:

BICEPS
BUILD BASEBALL SHAPED BICEPS

BUILD BASEBALL SHAPED BICEPS

06 BUILD BASEBALL SHAPED BICEPS

The biceps muscle has two heads. A short head, which is on the inside of the arm, and a long head, which is on the outside. This is the part that people see first. The main roll of the biceps is to flex the forearm, by bringing the hand towards the shoulder. In order to build powerful complete biceps, you need to learn that the biceps do not work by itself.

The brachialis, which is under the bicep when developed gives the bicep a larger and fuller appearance. Performing Isometric curls place undesirable tension on the tendon near the elbow. In other words, the biceps are placed in a very vulnerable position. Always maintain tension on the biceps and not the joint.

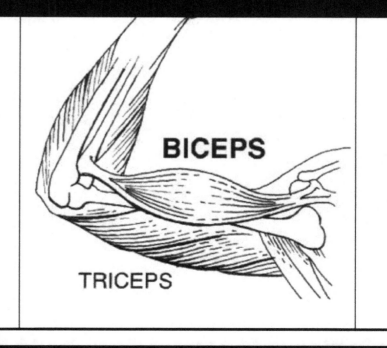

BICEPS

TRICEPS

BICEP EXERCISES

06 BUILD BASEBALL SHAPED BICEPS

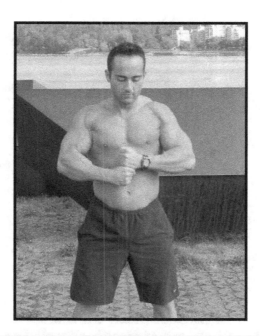

ISOMETRIC HAMMER CURLS

A great Bicep/Forearm combo. Place the wrists as shown in the picture above. Isometrically pull with bottom hand upwards while resisting with the top hand.

BICEP EXERCISES

06 BUILD BASEBALL SHAPED BICEPS

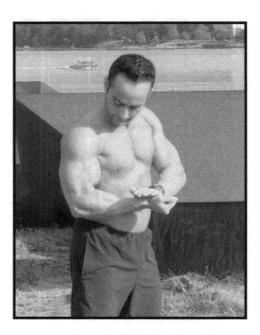

ISOMETRIC PALM UP CURLS

Grasp your right wrist with the left hand. Isometrically pull the right arm upward while resisting with the left hand.

BICEP EXERCISES

06 BUILD BASEBALL SHAPED BICEPS

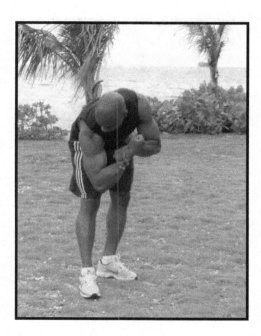

ISOMETRIC CONCENTRATION CURLS

This is a great bicep movement. Peak contraction to hit that long head again. As pictured in start position hold on to the right wrist with left hand. Isometrically pull the right arm while resisting with the left hand.

BICEP EXERCISES

06 BUILD BASEBALL SHAPED BICEPS

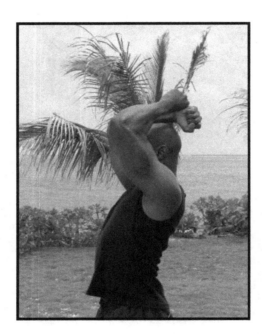

ISOMETRIC OVER-HEAD CURLS

Make a fist with both hands place it above your head. Isometrically pull the top fist downward while resisting with the bottom fist. Use a light to moderate tension due to the tricep tendons being quite sensitive at that position.

Chapter 7:

TRICEPS
DEVELOP POWERFUL TRICEPS

DEVELOP POWERFUL TRICEPS

07 DEVELOP POWERFUL TRICEPS

DEVELOP POWERFUL TRICEPS

The triceps has three heads: The lateral head, middle head and the long head. The role of the triceps is to straighten the arm. The triceps works in opposition to the biceps and brachialis muscles. The triceps has three heads this makes it much larger in mass than the biceps and the brachialis.

However unfortunately most pay attention to the biceps, leaving the triceps underdeveloped. The lateral head, which is on the outside is what people see first. The triceps are easy to develop and we have made it easy for the trainee to achieve this.

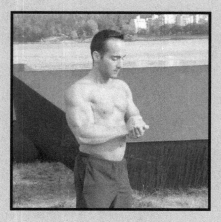

TRICEP EXERCISES

07 DEVELOP POWERFUL TRICEPS

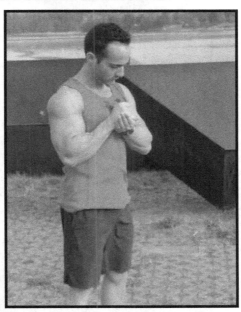

ISOMETRIC PUSHDOWNS

As shown above, Isometrically press the right arm forward while resisting with the left hand. Perform for desired seconds, then switch arms.

TRICEP EXERCISES

07 DEVELOP POWERFUL TRICEPS

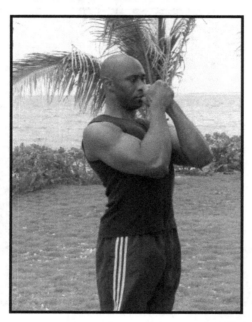

ISOMETRIC FORWARD EXTENSIONS

Place the left fist in the right hand. Isometrically push the left hand forward while resisting with the right hand.

TRICEP EXERCISES

07 DEVELOP POWERFUL TRICEPS

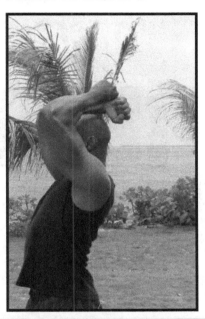

ISOMETRIC OVERHEAD EXTENSIONS

Make a fist with both hands place it as shown above. Isometrically push the bottom fist upward while resisting with the top fist. Use moderate tension due to the tricep tendons being quite sensitive at that position.

Chapter 8:

FOREARMS
DEVELOP RIPPED FOREARMS

DEVELOP RIPPED FOREARMS

08 DEVELOP RIPPED FOREARMS

DEVELOP RIPPED FOREARMS

DEVELOP RIPPED FOREARMS

Forearm muscles are involved in every daily activity, just like the calves and abdominals. We use these muscles all the time, when we drive, write, type, hold a bag and even open a door.

Many of the muscles of the forearm deal with Muscle-multi-use. When you are moving the elbow by lowering and raising the forearm. Moving the wrist up and down by, raising and lowering the hand. All Isometric exercises stress the forearms to contract which will increase your grip strength.

FOREARM EXERCISES

08 DEVELOP RIPPED FOREARMS

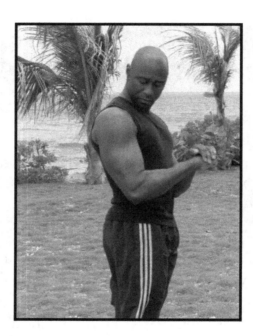

ISOMETRIC REVERSE CURLS

This is the Grand-daddy of all forearm exercises. A great bicep/ forearm widener. Place the left hand on top of the right fist. Isometrically pull the right hand upwards while resisting with the left hand.

Contract for desired seconds then switch arms. This exercise adds fullness to the upper arms giving the bicep a fuller appearance.

Chapter 9:

THIGHS
DEVELOP POWERFUL TIRELESS LEGS

DEVELOP POWERFUL TIRELESS LEGS

09 DEVELOP POWERFUL TIRELESS LEGS

DEVELOP POWERFUL THIGHS

The thigh muscles are basically made up of four main muscles: the vastus lateral muscle, this is located on the outside of the thighs. The vastus medial muscle, this is located on the inside of the thigh muscles towards the knee.

Better known as the tear drop because of its shape. The recus-femoris, which is located in the center of the muscles, and the vastus intermedius, this muscle is mostly covered by all the other muscles of the thighs. The Isometric Power Pulse Method will develop tireless thighs with a power pack punch.

LEG EXERCISES

09 DEVELOP POWERFUL TIRELESS LEGS

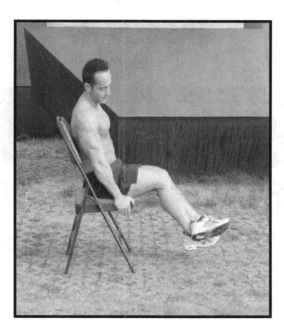

ISOMETRIC LEG EXTENSIONS

While seated on a chair, box or stool, place the right leg over the left as shown in the picture. Isometrically push the left leg outwards resisting with the right. Hold for desired seconds, then switch legs.

Chapter 9:

LOWER-BACK
DEVELOP POWERFUL LOWER BACK MUSCLES

DEVELOP POWERFUL LOWER BACK MUSCLES

09 DEVELOP POWERFUL LOWER BACK MUSCLES

POWERFUL LOWER BACK MUSCLES

Develop Powerful Lower back muscles
The lower back muscles support the lower part of the spine. When these muscles are well developed it builds a brace protecting the spine.

Apart from that the lower back muscles are responsible for bringing the body upright from a leaning forward position. Not only will the lower back be involved, but the glutes and hamstrings come into play as well.

LOWER BACK EXERCISES

09 DEVELOP POWERFUL LOWER BACK/HAMSTRINGS

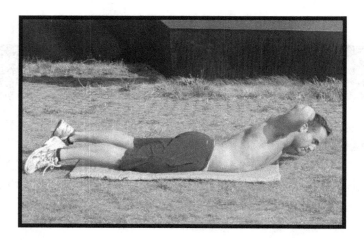

ISOMETRIC BACK EXTENSION

As shown above this is the finished position. Lay flat on the floor and perform this movement by raising the upper body upwards hold Isometrically at the top.

DEVELOP POWERFUL HAMSTRINGS

09 DEVELOP POWERFUL LOWER BACK/HAMSTRINGS

DEVELOP POWERFUL HAMSTRINGS

DEVELOP POWERFUL HAMSTRINGS

The hamstrings are the muscles at the back of the thighs.
These muscles are very powerful and work with the thigh muscles, hips, glutes and lower-back. The hamstrings are taxed in sporting activities, and although these muscles are not seen from the front they are often neglected.

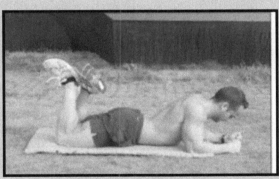

HAMSTRING CURLS

While on the stomach on the floor place the left leg over the right as shown, Isometrically pull the right leg upwards towards you while resisting with the left leg. Hold for desired seconds and switch legs.

Chapter 10:

CALVES
DEVELOP SHAPELY CALVES

DEVELOP SHAPELY CALVES

10 DEVELOP SHAPELY CALVES

DEVELOP SHAPELY CALVES

Develop shapely calves

The calves add a finished look to the lower leg with a diamond shape. This muscle has three heads (muscle parts) the soleus, this is under the large lateral head and gives the calves a full developed look viewed from the side and back.

The lateral and medial heads which are on the insides and in the middle of the muscle. The gastrocnemius make up the majority of the calf muscle. However, the longer the gastroc, the larger the potential for enhanced calf muscle development.

DEVELOP SHAPELY CALVES

10 DEVELOP SHAPELY CALVES

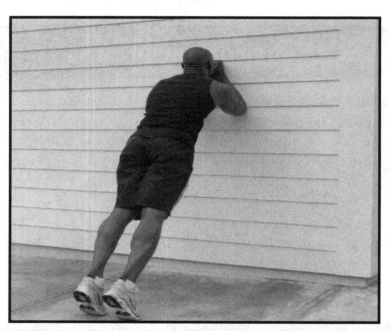

ISOMETRIC CONTRACTED RAISES

Stand at least 30 inches away from the wall, or position yourself as shown but make sure the calves are fully contracted and hold for desired seconds.

Chapter 11:

ABDOMINALS
DEVELOP RIPPED ABS

DEVELOP RIPPED ABS

11 DEVELOP RIPPED ABS

The abdominal muscles very important by revealing that the trainee has a lean physique. Plus the role of the abdominal muscles is to protect the spine. A lean chiseled set of abdominal muscles shows the opposite sex that the owner has a sign of virility.

Once these muscles are well developed this keeps the waist line and belly flat. There are various muscle structures that complete the overall look, the entire length of the abdominal wall, plus the internal and external obliques.

The lower sections of the abdominal muscles play the largest role in pro tecting the spine and storing belly fat. This is the easiest place for body fat to accumulate. Which makes training with self resistance the ideal exerciseto attack those muscle fibers to the maximum.

We cover the exercises that get the job done within this chapter.

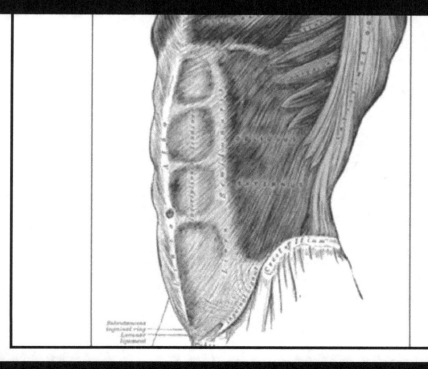

DEVELOP RIPPED ABS

11 DEVELOP RIPPED ABS

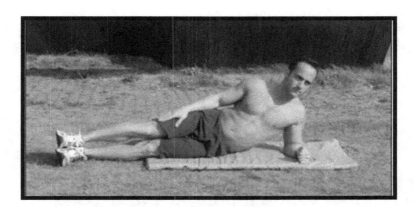

DEVELOP RIPPED ABDOMINALS

As noted in the introduction the abdominal wall includes four muscles: Let's cover the front first, which is the entire length from the chest to pubis is called the rectus abdominis, people simply say abs for short. The abdominal wall should be worked in three angles of flexion. The lower sections of the abdominal muscles. The upper sections of the abdominal wall, and the obliques. Which are rotator muscles.

DEVELOP RIPPED ABS

11 DEVELOP RIPPED ABS

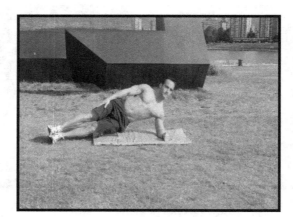

ISOMETRIC OBLIQUE HOLD

Normally people say I want to lose my love handles. Well rest assured this abdominal exercise really isolates the oblique muscles. These muscles supports the spine by making the abdominal wall more rigid.

Start off as shown above and hold the position for desired seconds. Then switch sides.

DEVELOP RIPPED ABS

11 DEVELOP RIPPED ABS

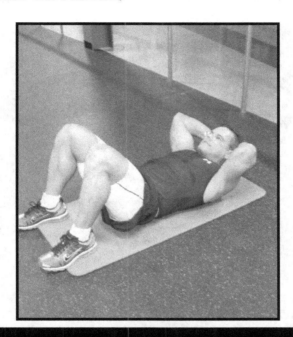

ISOMETRIC ABDOMINAL CRUNCH

Lay on your back. Place the hands at your ear, tilt your head back, focus on the ceiling and go into the upward position as shown. **HOLD ISOMETRICALLY AND DO NOT PULL ON THE HEAD.**

DEVELOP RIPPED ABS

11 DEVELOP RIPPED ABS

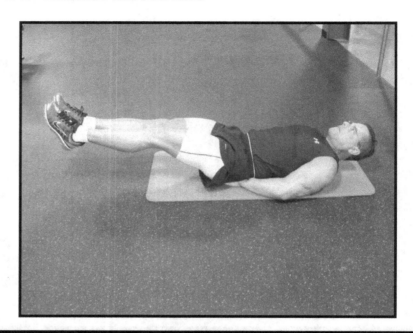

ISOMETRIC AB HOLD

As shown above, place your hands under your butt and hold the position Isometrically for the desired seconds. This exercise stimulates the entire abdominal wall.

Chapter 12:

ULTIMATE POWER PULSE METHOD

DEVELOP POWERFUL MUSCLES FAST

POWER PULSE

12 POWER PULSE

The Isometric Pulses is a slash between endurance-oriented fiber overload and a blood pooling element. There's various phases and multiple-holds times, that increases your strength, muscle size and build muscle density. The reason for this, is that most trainees are not activating the endurance components of the fast-twitch 2A fibers.

The best part about the Power Pulse Method, is that it stimulates the mito-chondria in the muscle cells. Plus the noncontractile proteins that do not directly contribute to the production of muscle force. This will begin to produce new muscle-growth and strength gains at a **FASTER** rate.

The reason the Power Pulse Method works like a charm is the endurance component effect. Longer load times, short rest between sets, and added fatigue accumulation. This form of training requires less force, but equals awesome hypertrophy pathways that build every facet of the muscle structure. So in short, you get larger muscles faster due to the mini-reps!

The Power Pulse Method have been tested on various subjects and it works **FAST**. Many would be skeptical with the higher hold times, However, in truth, we do not need ultra-high contractions to grow. We have been brainwashed into thinking heavy weights and High intensity Isometrics is the only way to an awesome body. Not any more.

In truth, we have a massive amount of predominance type 2A power endur-ance fibers. And the Power Pulses really stimulate and stress the sarcoplasm that gives the trainee a triple dose of increased muscle growth.
Isometric Power Pulses gets the job done in far less time. On top of that you will use various exercises to stimulate different fibers, this stimulate the bulk of the muscle for enhanced ongoing muscle-growth. Plus, muscle recruitment changes with each exercise and angle of pull. This promotes more growth.

POWER PULSE

12 POWER PULSE

We have the best exercises for enhancing muscle growth and strength for every body part. The Power Pulse Methods provide continuous tension on the working muscles that increase growth producing fiber expansion.

How does the Power Pulse Method works in building larger muscles? It is a spectacular muscle-producing plan because you are cramming a lot of contractions into a short amount of time. By performing Isometric mini-reps, followed by with a 5 second break between each round of reps pre-fatiguing the fibers for more growth activation within the upcoming pulsing reps and Isometric contractions.

This muscle building method is a serious **GET BIG** producing formula. The method works because it targets the motor units to perform extensive repetitive work. Along with an Isometric component tagged on. This creates unwanted irritation on the muscles being worked, and adaptation takes place where the muscles are forced to increase its size.

How do we perform the Power Pulse reps? Let's look at Phase one, using the chest press as an example.....Perform 20 Isometric 1 second mini-reps, followed by a 20 second Isometric contraction. Rest 5 seconds and repeat. This is a powerful muscle-producing-method and will really tax those 2A fast-twitch endurance fibers to the max. Okay, so now you understand the concept, it is time to build some serious muscle with Phase one of The Power Isometric Power Pulses.

POWER PULSE

12 POWER PULSE

My promise is that you will build every hypertrophic constituent to where your physique will become shredded, with eye-popping carved out muscle at every limb—and it will not take years to reach that goal. Trainees that carry out training with The Power Max Method will acheive pumped up muscles like never before. The restriction of blood flow to the muscles with enhanced tension times is painful but it works like magic.

Alot of nitric oxide is released within the system, which will dilate blood vessels in an attempt to overcome the decreased blood flow within the muscle fibers, this however activates growth hormone release.

All the added force increases in the sarcoplasmic fluid as it builds new and more efficient energy substrates and mitochondria to supercompensate for the oxygen debt from the extended set protocol. Muscular development is mostly the result of blood blockage (occlusion) and sarcoplasmic growth from the isometric holds and extended continuous-tension force.

That is why The Power Max muscle-program was developed. Moderate intensity loads is best for muscle growth triggers, along with an increase and special focus on the force output approach on the exercises. Extended-load time training with (medium-high intensity) for an extended set protocol, with no real rest between exercises is best to coax the muscle-building effect.

Cutting rest time between exercises has a large impact on the growth of the musculature. Once you follow the exercise protocol in this book you do not allow your muscles to recover between exercises, which will coax the release of growth hormone prompting, greater muscle growth. So in short, training the muscle in a fatigued state—with extended tension with a high amount of work, is the most efficient way to build larger stronger muscles faster.

POWER PULSE

12 POWER PULSE

This is why saraoplasmic wins due to the increase. However myofibrillar increases may be secondary here, but getting growth in the myofibrils will definetly add to a muscle's overall size. So, while sarcoplasmic increases is the primary growth factor in muscle tissue, it may be more true for some muscles than others.

Endurance-oriented muscle groups like forearms, abdominals, traps, hamstrings and calves respond best to sarcoplasmic stimulation in the majority of trainees. In most people, less-endurance-oriented muscle-groups require more of a balance of myofibrillar and sarcoplasmic stimulation to coax the greatest growth capacity. Nevertheless, with Power Pulses you will be training both "sides" of the type-2A fibers to achieve maximum muscle stimulation. So it is the time under load that governs optimal muscle-building size stimulation.

Thats why the Isometric Power Pulse Method is so effective. Tension time is enhanced and this creates drastic sarcoplasm stress for size increases and cause fatigue components for myofibrillar power stimulation. In simple terms, an extended exercise set primarily activates sarcoplasmic expansion. Which coax optimal size stimulation in both the myofibrils and sarcoplasm so you need to stimulate the two bases— tension/output for the myofibrils and extended load times for the sarcoplasm.

The extreme pump and burn indicates big sarcoplasmic-expansion effects. Thats why once the targeted muscle is under load for an extended period it will coax optimum sarcoplasmic stimulus, along with enhancing myofibrillar trauma and muscle-building growth activation. The bonus, is that the myofibrillar trauma also increases metabolic ramps that burns more bodyfat. So you get more muscular and leaner at the same time!

PHASE ONE

12 POWER X20

MONDAY, WEDNESDAY, FRIDAY (CHEST, BACK, MID-BACK, BICEPS, CALVES)
Perform 20 power pulses, followed by a 20 second Isometric hold, 3 sets each before moving to the next exercise.
Perform phase one for 2 weeks before moving to phase two.

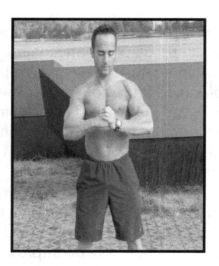
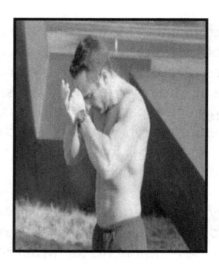
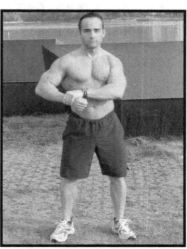
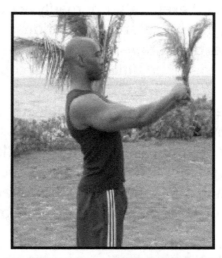

PHASE ONE

12 POWER X20

MONDAY, WEDNESDAY, FRIDAY
Routine continued.........

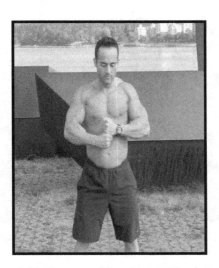
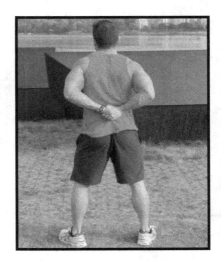
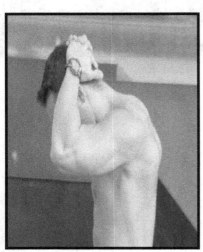
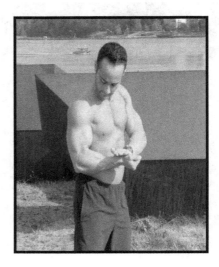

PHASE ONE

12 POWER X20

MONDAY, WEDNESDAY, FRIDAY
Routine continued...........

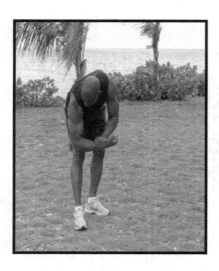 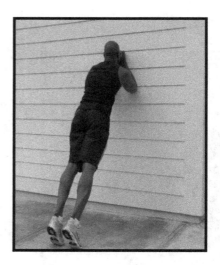

PHASE ONE MON, WED, FRI

PHASE ONE

12 POWER X20

TUESDAY, THURSDAY, SATURDAY (SHOULDERS, TRICEPS, THIGHS, HAMSTRINGS, ABS
Perform 20 power pulses, followed by a 20 second Isometric hold, 3 sets each before moving to the next exercise.
Perform phase one for 2 weeks before moving to phase two.

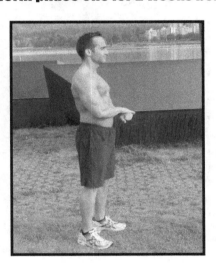
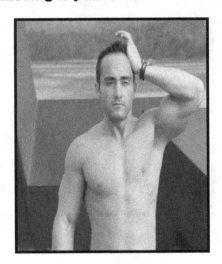

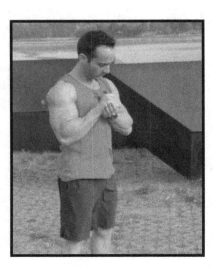
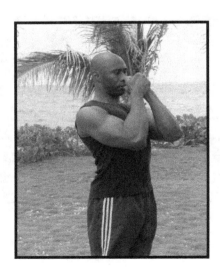

PHASE ONE

12 POWER X20

TUESDAY, THURSDAY, SATURDAY
Continued routine..........

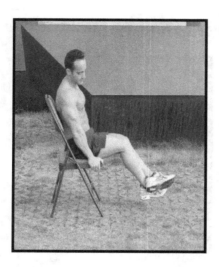
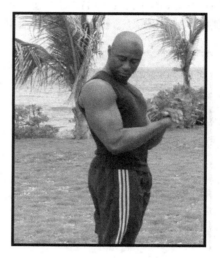

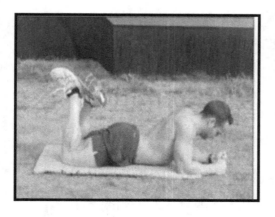
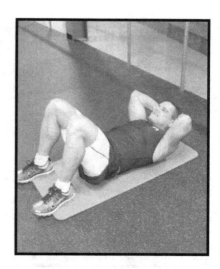

PHASE ONE

12 **POWER X20**

TUESDAY, THURSDAY, SATURDAY
Continued routine........

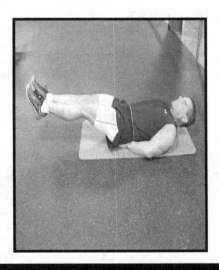 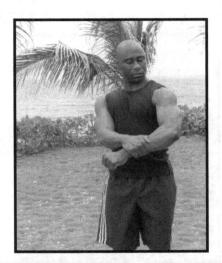

PHASE ONE TUES, THURS, SAT.

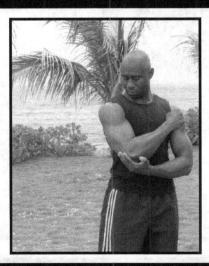

PHASE TWO

13 FAT-LOSS POWER MAX PROGRAM

MONDAY, WEDNESDAY, FRIDAY (BACK, ABS, LOWERBACK, CALVES, CHEST, SHOULDERS)
Within this phase perform the exercises on each page without rest until 5
rounds are completed. Perform 30 power pulses, followed by a 30 second
Isometric contraction. **Perform this routine for 2 weeks.**

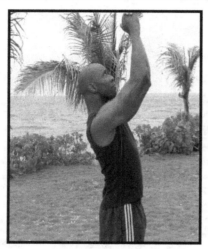

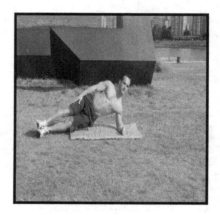

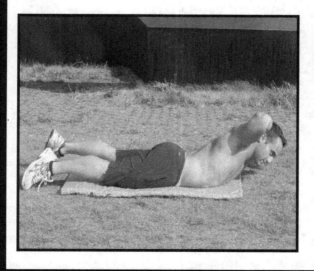

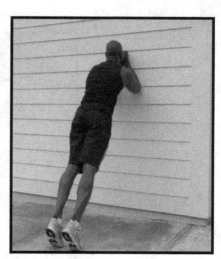

PHASE TWO

13 FAT-LOSS POWER MAX PROGRAM

MONDAY, WEDNESDAY, FRIDAY
Routine continued........

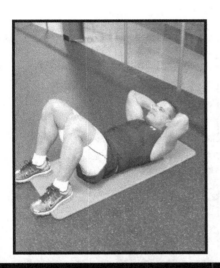 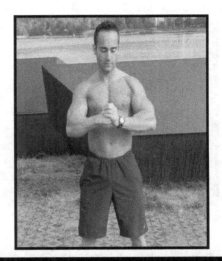

PHASE TWO   MON, WED, FRI.

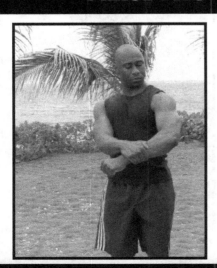 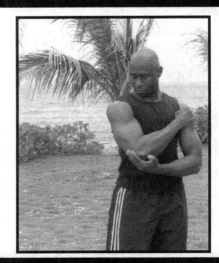

PHASE TWO

13 FAT-LOSS POWER MAX PROGRAM

TUESDAY, THURSDAY, SATURDAY (MID-BACK, BACK, BICEPS, TRICEPS, BACK, ABS)
Within this phase perform the exercises on each page without rest until 5 rounds are completed. Perform 30 power pulses, followed by a 30 second Isometric contraction. **Perform this routine for 2 weeks.**

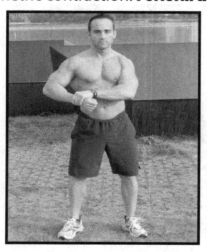
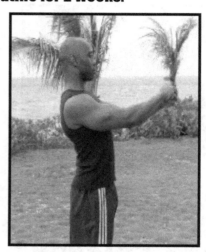

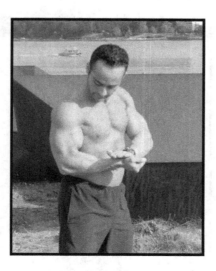
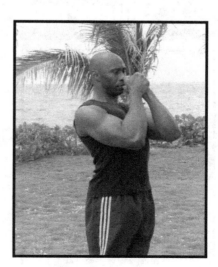

PHASE TWO

13 FAT-LOSS POWER MAX PROGRAM

TUESDAY, THURSDAY, SATURDAY
Routine continued..........

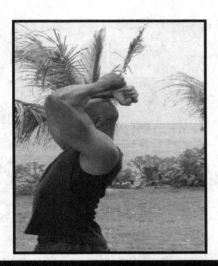
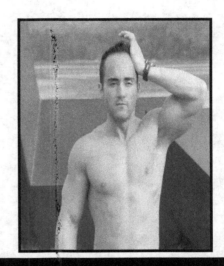

PHASE TWO   TUES, THURS, SAT.

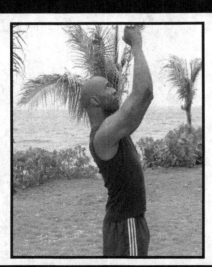
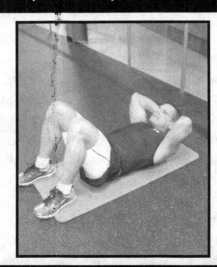

ENHANCING MUSCLE FIBER ACTIVATION

14 MUSCLE BUILDING ACCELERATION PROGRAM

Enhancing-Muscle-Fiber-Activation

The first thing The Power Pulse Method will address is the understanding of how to irritate and coax muscle growth and strength with the Muscle-Building-master-plan of muscle-fiber-stimulation.

Type 1s Are aerobic, and require oxygen to fire, it contains loads of mitochondria, where fat is burned for energy. With our program you will call on these fibers a lot!

Type 2As Have both aerobic and anaerobic components. You will use these for low-contraction isometric work. Mitochondria is present, but far fewer than the type 1s.

In all truth, these fiber types fire on a multi-extending set principle, but at different capacities. So, the harder the contraction, the less your type1s come into play. So on extreme force with strength-building Isometric contractions, (which I do not recommend) very few type 1s fire; however, ultra-heavy isometric contractions is not the best way to create and coax muscle size and strength gains. The reason...

The trainee need increased time under load to coax the muscle fibers to grow, so in truth trainees need to emphasize the endurance-fast-twitch-fibers to increase muscle size and strength. If you're looking for increased muscle growth, medium intensity contractions will get the job done safely and effectively.

By combining the various tension times within the upcoming phases you will train all facets of the muscle for optimal development and strength.

This book shows you how to perform these simple and unique exercises safely and effectively, by increasing the (myofibrils) and the more endurance part (sarcoplasm), not to mention the type-1 aerobic fibers.

ENHANCING MUSCLE FIBER ACTIVATION

14 MUSCLE BUILDING ACCELERATION PROGRAM

Enhancing-Muscle-Fiber-Activation

It has been suggested that Isometrics need to be performed at high intensities for low second holds that proclaim is the key to optimum muscle growth and strength. That is not 100 percent accurate; you see, most recommend trainees perform a 5-10 second isometric static hold. If they do this, the target muscle is only under tension for a short time. This is not an effective way to get ripped, increase muscle size or maintain healthy joints, by using that time under load frame, lots of sarcoplasmic "endurance" growth potential effects are left out.

You want both medium and longer tension times for optimum muscle-building-stimulation, which can be achieved with various contractions in the 30 plus second range, or tension that last up to 60-plus seconds, for 2A sarcoplasmic expansion + endurance power type-1 activation along with safe tendon strengthening.

Using the methods within these pages with moderate tension will build up more muscle strength with healthy tendons, than people that train in the traditional way of high resistance. Performing the contractions with moderate resistance will result in leaner, stronger and bigger muscles for life..

The reason being, with moderate tension sets the trainee can fatigue the endurance slow-twitch fibers, with more precision at the beginning of the extended set. This forces more endurance fast-twitch fibers to fire after 40 plus seconds, exactly what you need to coax more muscle. Okay, so now you under stand the extended set muscle-enhancing method.

ENHANCING MUSCLE FIBER ACTIVATION

14 MUSCLE BUILDING ACCELERATION PROGRAM

The "Extended Power Pump" extention for Quality Muscle

What is the ideal time under tension isometric hold for increasing sculpted muscle-gains? In all truth, doing sets with 30 plus extended holds in a few phases gets the muscle-building job done. It's a special blow-torch Isometric Power phase which, will produce increased hardening and will induce the fat-burning process along with increasing an amazing pump to coax muscle-building-gains.

Now why is it by doing extended-endurance-type isometric holds build lean muscle and increases strength gains more effectively? Because, it causes more intense contractions to the targeted muscle fibers more times over than so-called "traditional" isometric holds, this increases greater degrees of protein remodeling in the targeted muscles.

So in other words, the extended tension times cause more muscle irritation, which activates significantly more endurance-fast-twitch power fibers. We are forced to believe that intense powerful isometric holds of 5-10 seconds will forge the best gains—NO. Doing high tension isometric holds will lead to tendon damage and muscle strain.

ENHANCING MUSCLE FIBER ACTIVATION

14 MUSCLE BUILDING ACCELERATION PROGRAM

What is a Self-resistance-Isometric contraction

An Isometric contraction is where the trainee apply force and hold that contraction by maintaining a static position. This increases tension (force out put) on the muscle fibers to promote muscular tension which produce muscle size and strength gains.

A classic example is shown in the picture below by placing the hands at chest level and pressing the palms together holding the contraction for seconds at a time. Please note while performing all of the Isometric exercises it is important that you breathe normal. **DO NOT HOLD YOUR BREATH**

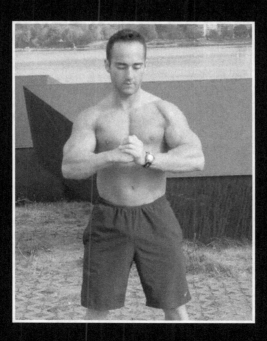

Chapter 14:

ENHANCING MUSCLE FIBER ACTIVATION

MUSCLE ACCELERATION PROGRAMS
ISOMETRIC HOLDS VARY DURING THE WEEK

ENHANCING MUSCLE FIBER ACTIVATION

14 MUSCLE ACCELERATION PROGRAM

HOW TO PERFORM THIS ROUTINE:

Perform a 20 second Isometric contraction. At 20 seconds, perform 30 power pulses, along with another 20 second Isometric hold. Rest 15 seconds between sets. **Two work sets each exercise, perform this program for 3 weeks.**

DAY ONE

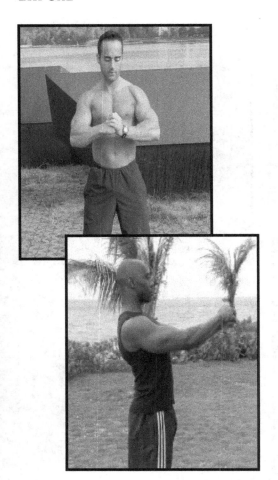

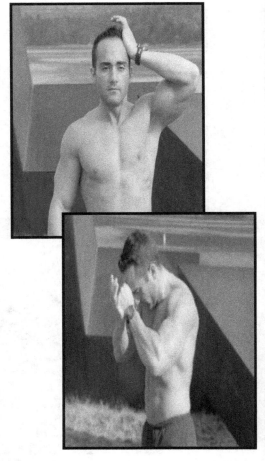

ENHANCING MUSCLE FIBER ACTIVATION

14 MUSCLE ACCELERATION PROGRAM

HOW TO PERFORM THIS ROUTINE:

Perform a 20 second Isometric contraction. At 20 seconds, perform 30 power pulses, along with another 20 second Isometric hold. Rest 15 seconds between sets.

DAY ONE continued..........

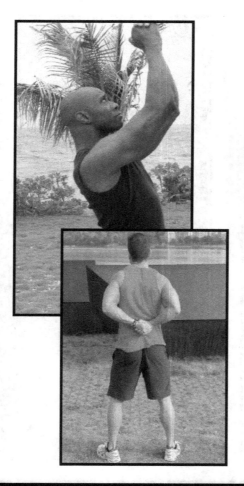

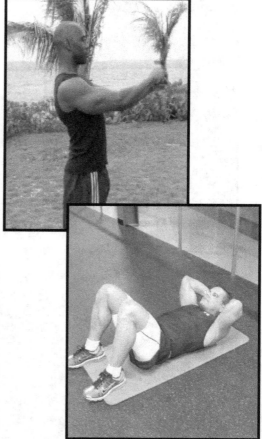

ENHANCING MUSCLE FIBER ACTIVATION

14 MUSCLE ACCELERATION PROGRAM

HOW TO PERFORM THIS ROUTINE:

Perform a 30 second Isometric contraction. At 30 seconds, perform 20 power pulses, along with another 30 second Isometric hold. Rest 15 seconds between sets. **Two-three work sets per exercise.**

DAY TWO

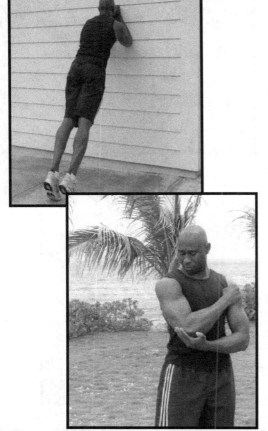

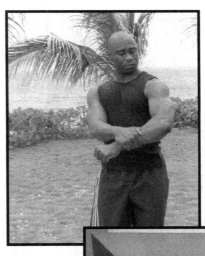

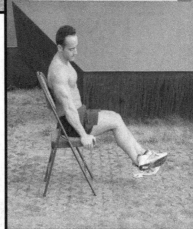

ENHANCING MUSCLE FIBER ACTIVATION

14 MUSCLE ACCELERATION PROGRAM

HOW TO PERFORM THIS ROUTINE:

Perform a 30 second Isometric contraction. At 30 seconds, perform 20 power pulses, along with another 30 second Isometric hold. Rest 15 seconds between sets. **Two-three work sets per exercise.**

DAY TWO continued............

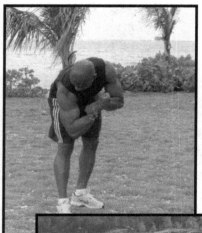

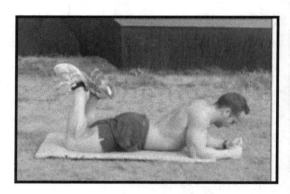

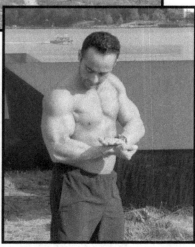

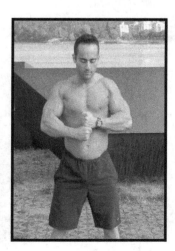

ENHANCING MUSCLE FIBER ACTIVATION

14 MUSCLE ACCELERATION PROGRAM

HOW TO PERFORM THIS ROUTINE:

Perform 10 Isometric Pulses. On your 10th rep perform a 20 second isometric contraction. Perform 3 sets each exercise, rest 5 seconds between sets.

DAY THREE

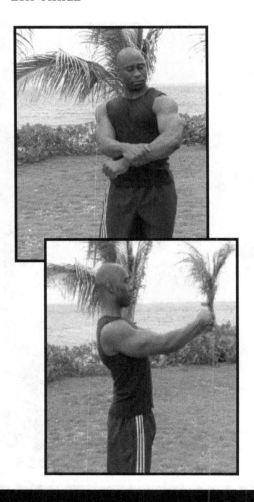

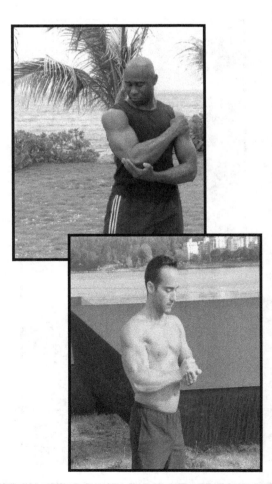

ENHANCING MUSCLE FIBER ACTIVATION

14 MUSCLE ACCELERATION PROGRAM

HOW TO PERFORM THIS ROUTINE:

Perform 10 Isometric Pulses. On your 10th rep perform a 20 second isometric contraction. Perform 3 sets each exercise, rest 5 seconds between sets.

DAY THREE continued.......

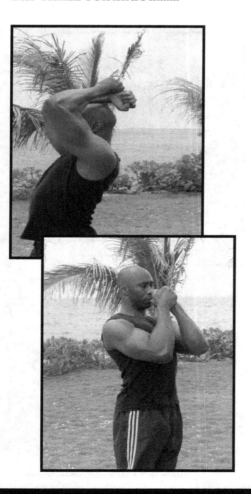

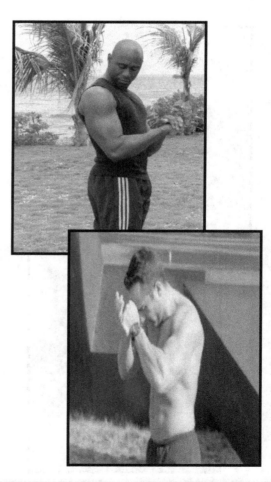

ENHANCING MUSCLE FIBER ACTIVATION

14 MUSCLE ACCELERATION PROGRAM

HOW TO PERFORM THIS ROUTINE:

Perform 10 Isometric Pulses. On your 10th rep perform a 20 second isometric contraction. Perform 3 sets each exercise, rest 5 seconds between sets.

DAY THREE continued.......

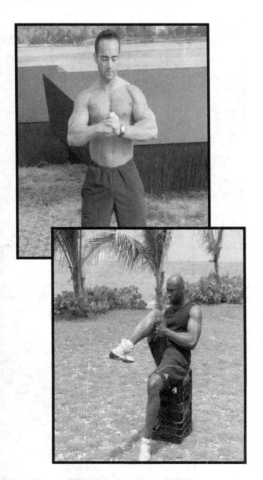

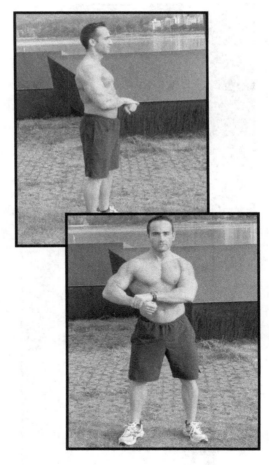

ENHANCING MUSCLE FIBER ACTIVATION

14 MUSCLE ACCELERATION PROGRAM

HOW TO PERFORM THIS ROUTINE:

Perform 40 Isometric pulses, on your 40th rep perform a 20 second isometric contraction. Perform 3 sets each exercise, resting 10 seconds between sets.

DAY FOUR

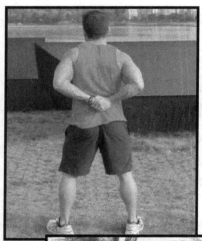
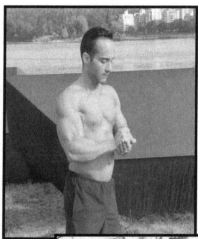
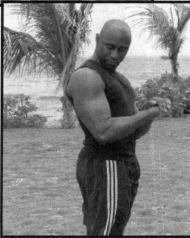
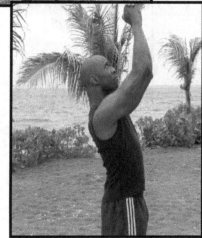

ENHANCING MUSCLE FIBER ACTIVATION

14 MUSCLE ACCELERATION PROGRAM

HOW TO PERFORM THIS ROUTINE:

Perform 40 Isometric pulses, on your 40th rep perform a 20 second isometric contraction. Perform 3 sets each exercise, resting 10 seconds between sets.

DAY FOUR continued......

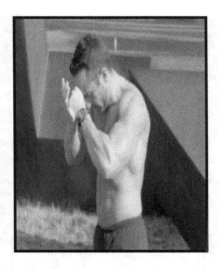

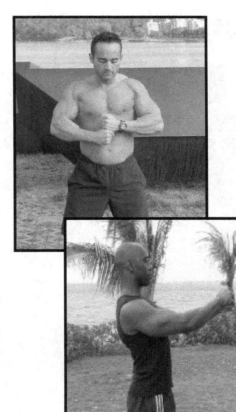

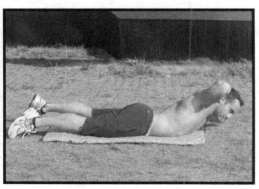

ENHANCING MUSCLE FIBER ACTIVATION

14 MUSCLE ACCELERATION PROGRAM

HOW TO PERFORM THIS ROUTINE:

Perform a 60 second isometric contraction. Perform 4 sets each exercise, rest
ing 5 seconds between sets.

DAY FIVE

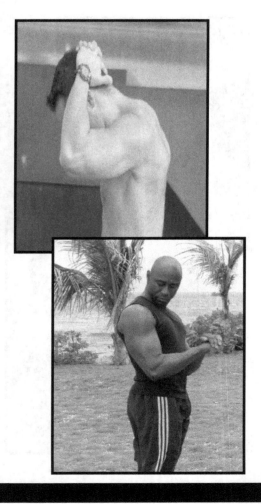

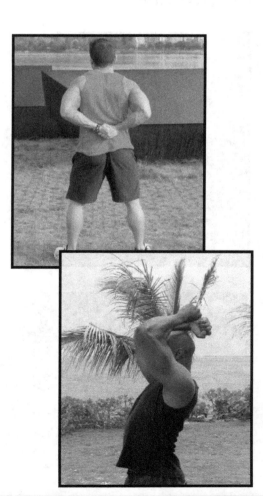

ENHANCING MUSCLE FIBER ACTIVATION

14 MUSCLE ACCELERATION PROGRAM

HOW TO PERFORM THIS ROUTINE:
Perform a 60 second isometric contraction. Perform 4 sets each exercise, resting 5 seconds between sets.

DAY FIVE continued.....

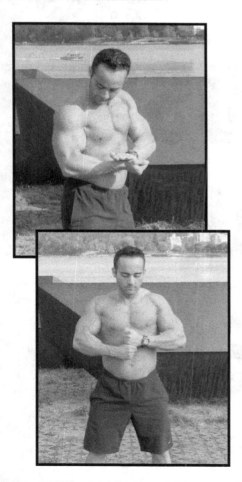
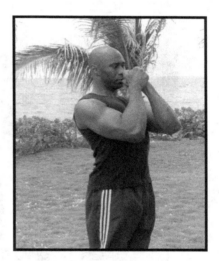
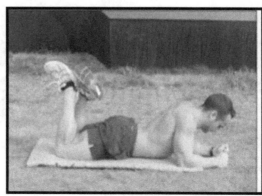

Chapter 15:

THE ISOMETRIC FAT-LOSS PLAN PHASE ONE

THE ISOMETRIC FAT-LOSS PLAN

15 FAT-LOSS PLAN

THE ISOMETRIC FAT-LOSS "GET RIPPED PHASE"

Phase 1: In this phase —you crank out various power pulses and Isometric contractions throughout the week. This extended load time activates higher percentages of fast-twitch fibers, so it is one of the best growth-fiber-activating phases.

Phase 2: In this phase—perform a 40 second Isometric contraction per exercise. This fatigues those last remaining fast-twitch fibers, pushing the muscle fibers past the growth threshold.

Phase 3: In this phase—perform a 60 second Isometric contraction, followed by 30 power pulses per exercise. This increases muscle size by increasing fiber expansion and growth hormone release due to the burning effect.

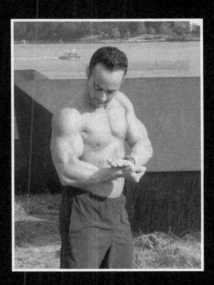

PHASE ONE

15 THE ISOMETRIC FAT-LOSS PLAN

HOW TO PERFORM THIS ROUTINE:
PHASE ONE
Perform 40 power pulses, followed by a 20 second Isometric contraction each exercise.....2-3 sets

DAY ONE

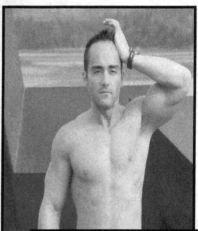
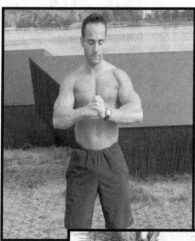
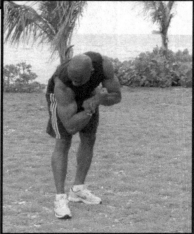
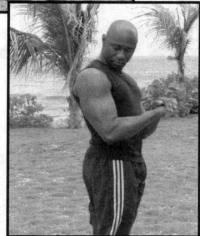

PHASE ONE

15 ISOMETRIC FAT-LOSS PLAN

HOW TO PERFORM THIS ROUTINE:
PHASE ONE

Perform 40 power pulses, followed by a 20 second Isometric contraction each exercise.....2-3 sets

DAY ONE continued.............

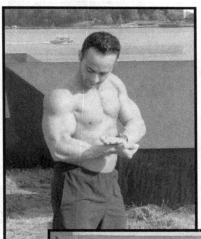
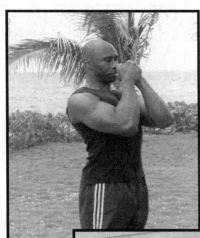
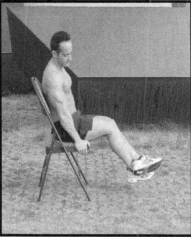
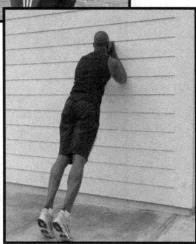

PHASE ONE

15 THE ISOMETRIC FAT-LOSS PLAN

HOW TO PERFORM THIS ROUTINE:
PHASE ONE

Perform 20 power pulses, followed by a 30 second Isometric contraction each exercise.....2-3 sets

DAY TWO

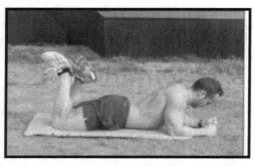

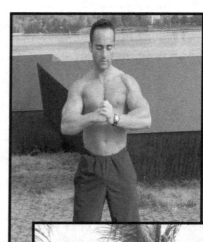

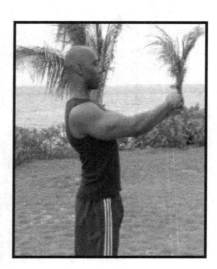

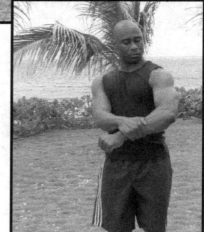

PHASE ONE

15 THE ISOMETRIC FAT-LOSS PLAN

HOW TO PERFORM THIS ROUTINE:
PHASE ONE
Perform 20 power pulses, followed by a 30 second Isometric contraction each exercise.....2-3 sets

DAY TWO continued.......

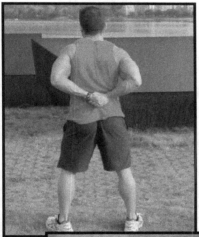

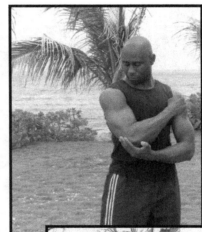

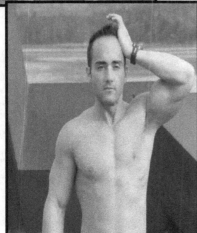

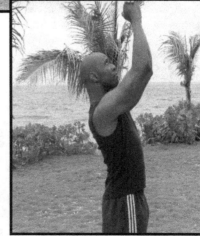

PHASE ONE

15 THE ISOMETRIC FAT-LOSS PLAN

HOW TO PERFORM THIS ROUTINE:
PHASE ONE

Perform 40 power pulses, followed by a 20 second Isometric contraction each exercise.....2 sets

DAY THREE

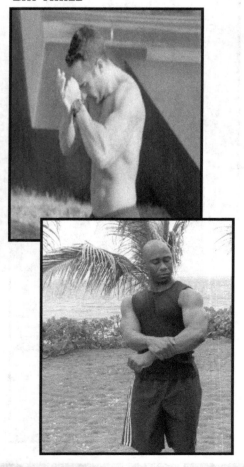

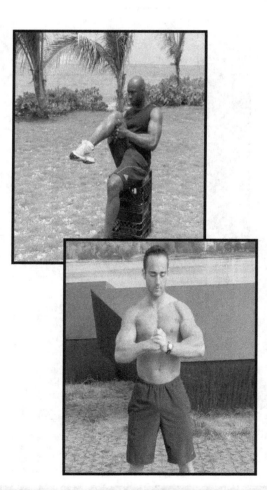

PHASE ONE

15 THE ISOMETRIC FAT-LOSS PLAN

HOW TO PERFORM THIS ROUTINE:
PHASE ONE

Perform 40 power pulses, followed by a 20 second Isometric contraction each exercise.....2 sets

DAY THREE continued..........

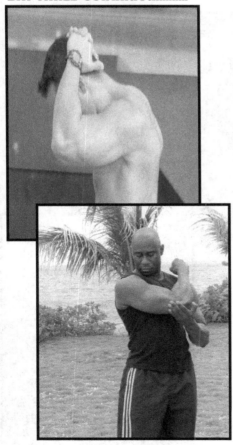
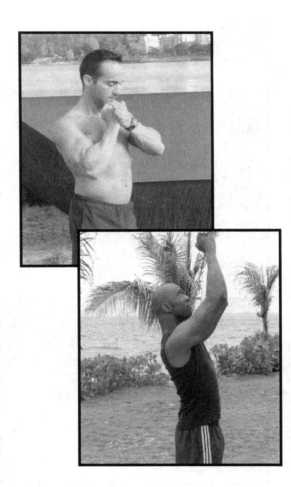

PHASE ONE

15 THE ISOMETRIC FAT-LOSS PLAN

HOW TO PERFORM THIS ROUTINE:
PHASE ONE

Perform 25 power pulses, followed by a 30 second Isometric contraction each exercise.....2 sets

DAY FOUR

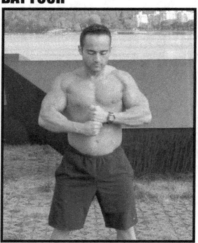

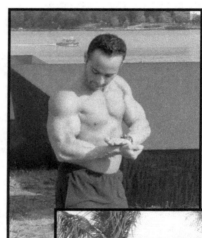

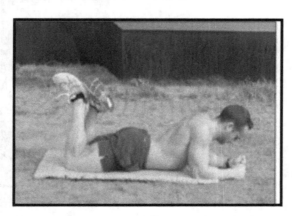

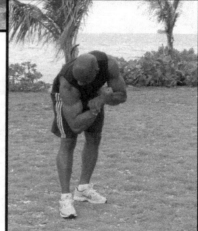

PHASE ONE

15 THE ISOMETRIC FAT-LOSS PLAN

HOW TO PERFORM THIS ROUTINE:
PHASE ONE

Perform 25 power pulses, followed by a 30 second Isometric contraction each exercise.....2 sets

DAY FOUR continued...........

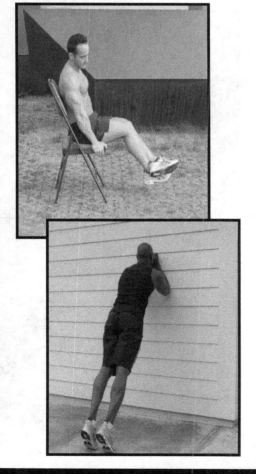

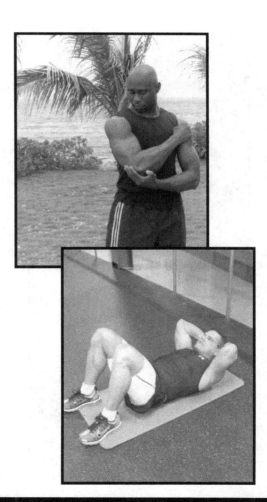

PHASE ONE

15 THE ISOMETRIC FAT-LOSS PLAN

HOW TO PERFORM THIS ROUTINE:
PHASE ONE

Perform 40 power pulses, followed by a 20 second Isometric contraction each exercise.....2 sets

DAY FIVE

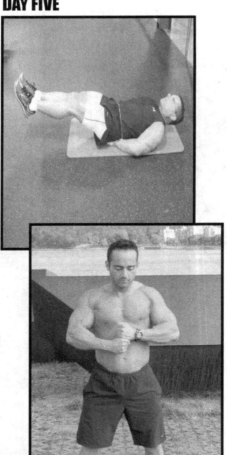

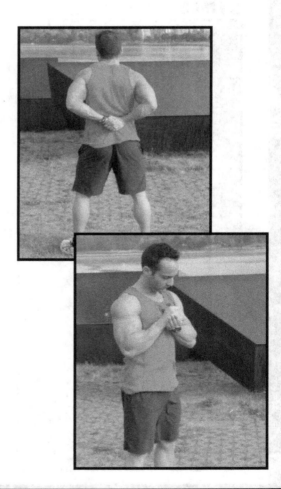

PHASE ONE

15 THE ISOMETRIC FAT-LOSS PLAN

HOW TO PERFORM THIS ROUTINE:
PHASE ONE
Perform 40 power pulses, followed by a 20 second Isometric contraction each exercise.....2 sets

DAY FIVE continued.............

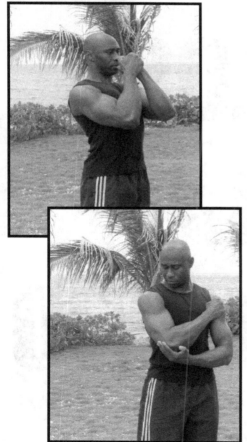

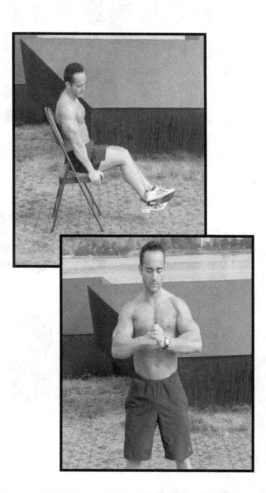

Chapter 15:

THE ISOMETRIC FAT-LOSS PLAN PHASE TWO

PHASE TWO

15 THE ISOMETRIC FAT-LOSS PLAN

HOW TO PERFORM THIS ROUTINE:
PHASE TWO

Perform a 40 second Isometric contraction each exercise.....4 sets each exercise. **Alternate Day one and Day two for 6 days straight.**

DAY ONE

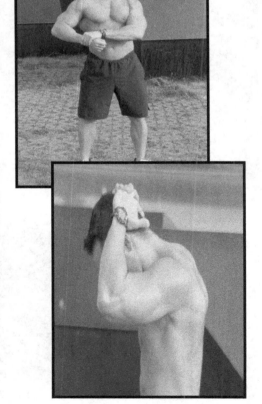
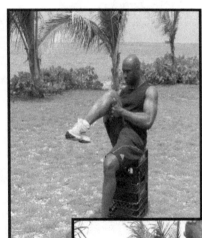
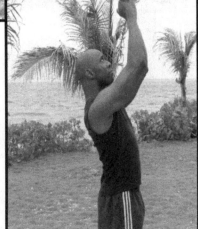

PHASE TWO

15 THE ISOMETRIC FAT-LOSS PLAN

HOW TO PERFORM THIS ROUTINE:
PHASE TWO

Perform a 40 second Isometric contraction each exercise.....4 sets each exercise.

DAY ONE continued..........

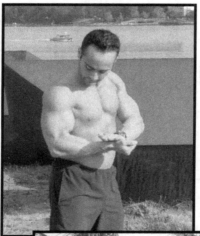

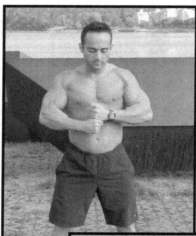

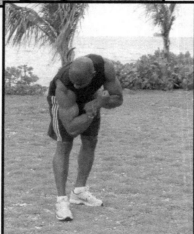

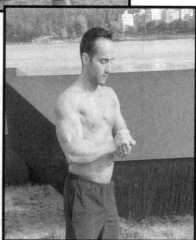

PHASE TWO

15 THE ISOMETRIC FAT-LOSS PLAN

HOW TO PERFORM THIS ROUTINE:
PHASE TWO

Perform a 40 second Isometric contraction each exercise.....4 sets each exercise.

DAY TWO

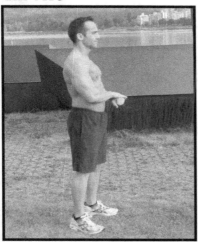
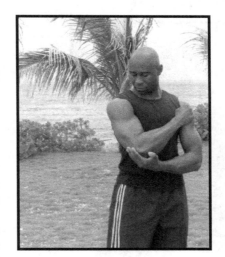

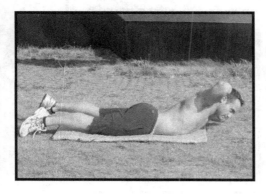
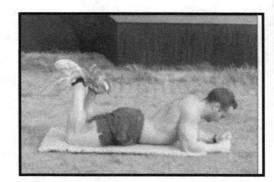

PHASE TWO

15 THE ISOMETRIC FAT-LOSS PLAN

HOW TO PERFORM THIS ROUTINE:
PHASE TWO

Perform a 40 second Isometric contraction each exercise.....4 sets each exercise.

DAY TWO continued........

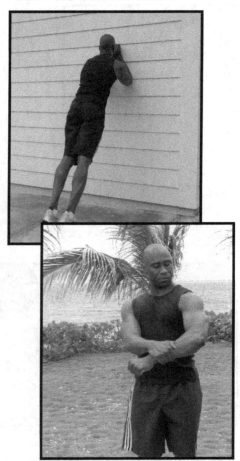

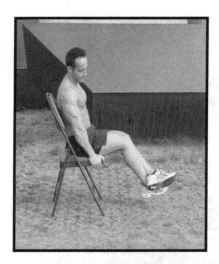

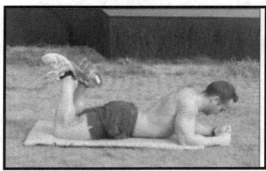

Chapter 15:

THE ISOMETRIC FAT-LOSS PLAN PHASE THREE

PHASE THREE

15 THE ISOMETRIC FAT-LOSS PLAN

HOW TO PERFORM THIS ROUTINE:
PHASE THREE

Perform a 60 second Isometric contraction, followed by a 30 second Isometric pulses each exercise.....4 sets.

DAY ONE

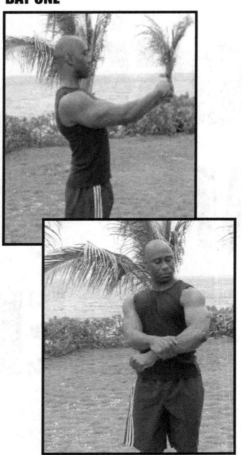

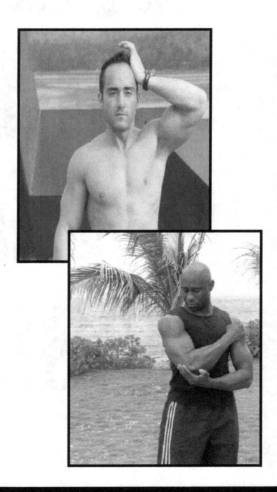

PHASE THREE

15 THE ISOMETRIC FAT-LOSS PLAN

HOW TO PERFORM THIS ROUTINE:
PHASE THREE

Perform a 60 second Isometric contraction, followed by a 30 second Isometric pulses each exercise.....4 sets.

DAY ONE continued...........

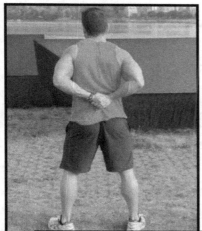

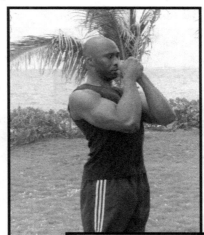

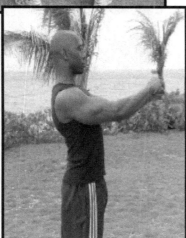

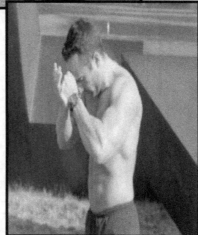

PHASE THREE

15 THE ISOMETRIC FAT-LOSS PLAN

HOW TO PERFORM THIS ROUTINE:
PHASE THREE

Perform a 60 second Isometric contraction, followed by a 30 second Isometric pulses. Perform 4 sets.

DAY TWO

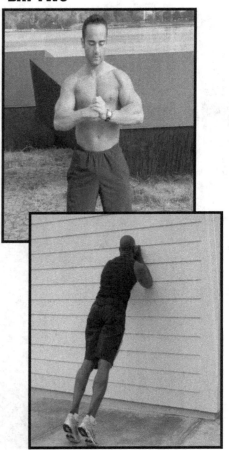

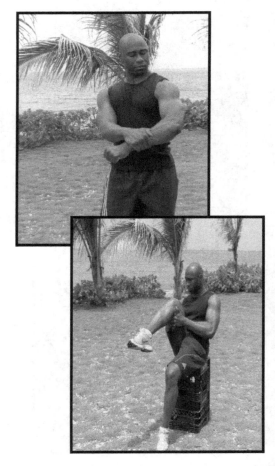

PHASE THREE

15 THE ISOMETRIC FAT-LOSS PLAN

HOW TO PERFORM THIS ROUTINE:
PHASE THREE
Perform a 60 second Isometric contraction, followed by a 30 second Isometric pulses each exercise.....4 sets.

DAY TWO continued...........

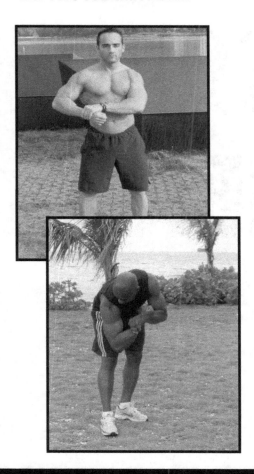

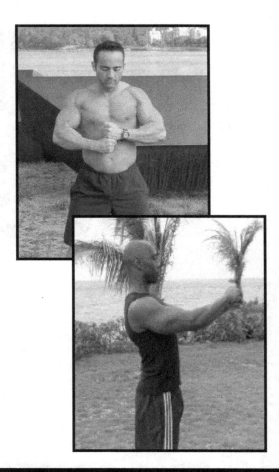

Chapter 16

THE ISOMETRIC POWER 10 PROGRAM

POWER 10

16 THE ISOMETRIC POWER 10 PROGRAM

THE ISOMETRIC POWER 10 PROGRAM

The Isometric Power 10 Program is a great multi-angular strength-enhancing system. Below is a great program The Isometric 10,10,10 Program.
This is were you hammer your muscles non-stop for an intense fat burning trigger. How does this program burn bodyfat and increase lean muscle size?

As a result of these routines, in short, the trainee will move quickly from exercise to exercise with no rest between exercises to highten extreme fiber stimulation and increase fat-burning-hormonal release. Which is a fiber-activation growth enhancer. This method of extended-time under load sets coax additional growth fibers to fire rapidly within the contraction being held.

Below The Isometric 10,10,10 Program for each target muscle will host exercises to stimulate full Flexion and contractability. However the trainee will receive maximum muscle fiber and tendon stimulation with this Isometric Program. How do you perform the program? Perform 10 second power pulses rest 5 seconds, perform another 10 more pulses, rest 5 seconds, then perform a 10 second Isometric contraction. Thats one set.

POWER 10

16 THE ISOMETRIC POWER 10 PROGRAM

HOW TO PERFORM THIS ROUTINE:
THE ISOMETRIC FAT LOSS PROGRAM

Perform this **ISOMETRIC WORKOUT**—by placing the muscle at the contracted position. Perform10 power pulses, relax for 5 seconds, perform another 10 pulses, relax for 5 seconds, then perform a 10 second Isometric contraction. Perform all exercises without rest. Perform 3 rounds

Alternate day one and day two for 6 days per week.
DAY ONE

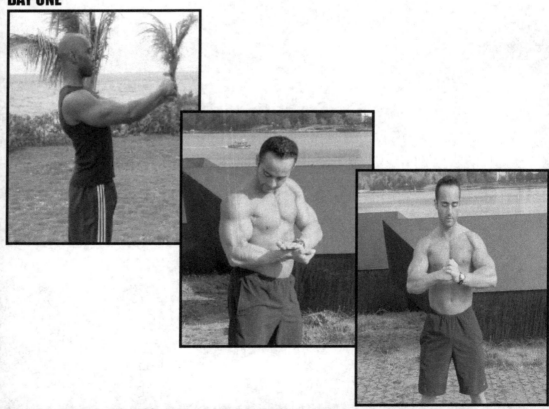

POWER 10

16 THE ISOMETRIC POWER 10 PROGRAM

HOW TO PERFORM THIS ROUTINE:
THE ISOMETRIC FAT LOSS PROGRAM

Perform this **ISOMETRIC WORKOUT**—by placing the muscle at the contracted position. Perform10 power pulses, relax for 5 seconds, perform another 10 pulses, relax for 5 seconds, then perform a 10 second Isometric contraction. Perform all exercises without rest. Perform 3 rounds

DAY ONE continued..........

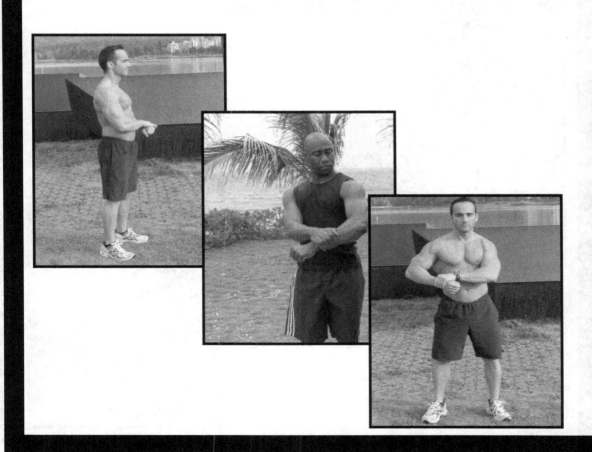

POWER 10

16 THE ISOMETRIC POWER 10 PROGRAM

HOW TO PERFORM THIS ROUTINE:
THE ISOMETRIC FAT LOSS PROGRAM

Perform this **ISOMETRIC WORKOUT**—by placing the muscle at the contracted position. Perform10 power pulses, relax for 5 seconds, perform another 10 pulses, relax for 5 seconds, then perform a 10 second Isometric contraction. Perform all exercises without rest. Perform 3 rounds

Alternate day one and day two for 6 days per week.
DAY ONE continued......

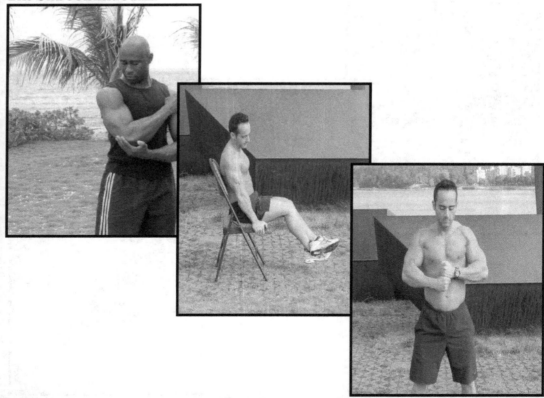

POWER 10

16 THE ISOMETRIC POWER 10 PROGRAM

HOW TO PERFORM THIS ROUTINE:
THE ISOMETRIC FAT LOSS PROGRAM

Perform this **ISOMETRIC WORKOUT**—by placing the muscle at the contracted position. Perform 10 power pulses, relax for 5 seconds, perform another 10 pulses, relax for 5 seconds, then perform a 10 second Isometric contraction. Perform all exercises without rest. Perform 3 rounds

Alternate day one and day two for 6 days per week.
DAY TWO

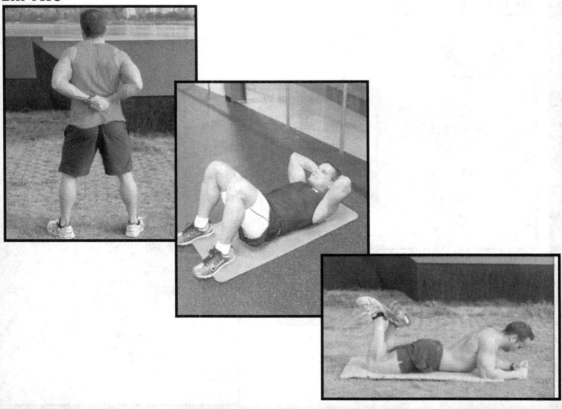

POWER 10

16 THE ISOMETRIC POWER 10 PROGRAM

HOW TO PERFORM THIS ROUTINE:
THE ISOMETRIC FAT LOSS PROGRAM

Perform this **ISOMETRIC WORKOUT**—by placing the muscle at the contracted position. Perform 10 power pulses, relax for 5 seconds, perform another 10 pulses, relax for 5 seconds, then perform a 10 second Isometric contraction. Perform all exercises without rest. Perform 3 rounds

**Alternate day one and day two for 6 days per week.
DAY TWO continue........**

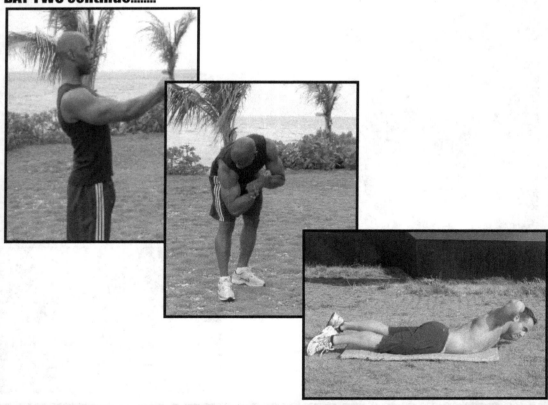

POWER 10

16 THE ISOMETRIC PIOWER 10 PROGRAM

HOW TO PERFORM THIS ROUTINE:
THE ISOMETRIC FAT LOSS PROGRAM

Perform this **ISOMETRIC WORKOUT**—by placing the muscle at the contracted position. Perform 10 power pulses, relax for 5 seconds, perform another 10 pulses, relax for 5 seconds, then perform a 10 second Isometric contraction. Perform all exercises without rest. Perform 3 rounds

Alternate day one and day two for 6 days per week.
DAY TWO continued...........

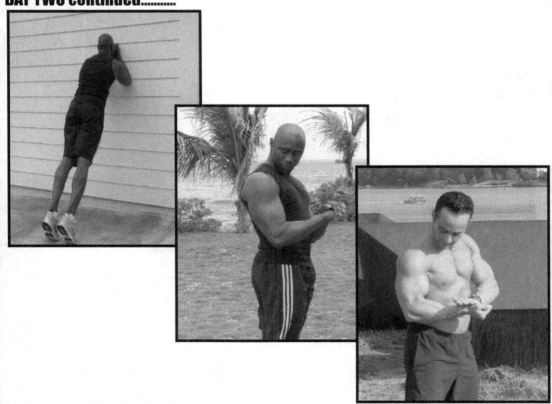

POWER 10

16 THE ISOMETRIC POWER 10 PROGRAM

HOW TO PERFORM THIS ROUTINE:
THE ISOMETRIC FAT LOSS PROGRAM

Perform this **ISOMETRIC WORKOUT**—by placing the muscle at the contracted position. Perform10 power pulses, relax for 5 seconds, perform another 10 pulses, relax for 5 seconds, then perform a 10 second Isometric contraction. Perform all exercises without rest. Perform 3 rounds

Alternate day one and day two for 6 days per week.
DAY TWO continued...........

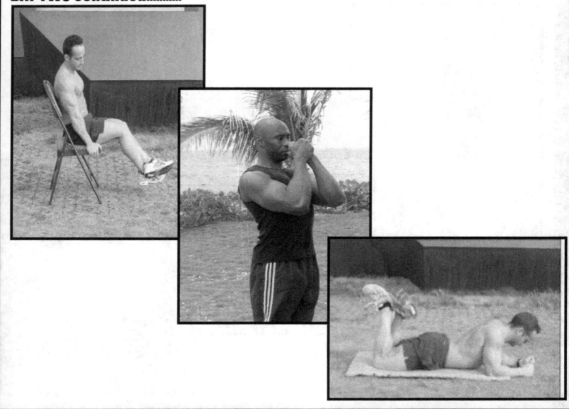

Chapter 17

THE ISOMETRIC POWER PULSE X 40 PROGRAM

THE ISOMETRIC POWER PULSE X40 PROGRAM

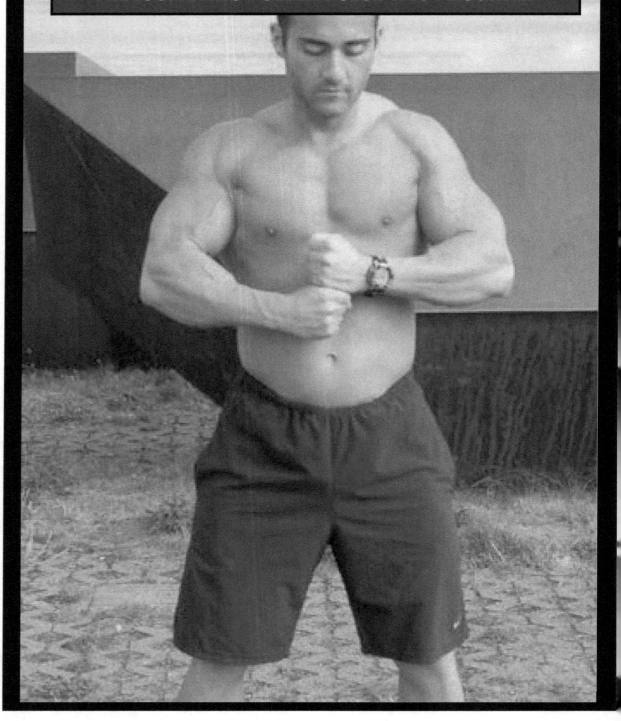

THE ISOMETRIC POWER PULSE X40 PROGRAM

17 POWER PULSE X40

The Isometric Power Pulse x40 Program is an awesome size and defination enhancer. The trainee can perform loads of mini-contractions in a short space of time—and the first few mini-reps do a great job of fatiguing the slow-twitch fibers for more growth-fiber activation on the following reps to follow. All it takes is two to three rounds, that's a serious muscle-building routine; and it should take you less than 20 minutes. This routine muscle blast increases the pump in the fibers while burning bodyfat **FAST**.

The trainee is also cranking out a lot of reps in a short space of time, but the sets go from ridiculously easy feeling (for cumulative slow-twitch fatigue) to some of the most intense full blown pumps you've ever done this really stimulates (growth-fiber-activation). The key is the intense short mini-contraction reps that lasts between 1-2 seconds per contraction this adds cumulative fatigue, as well as volume. The pump will be super crazy and off the charts.

Here's how it is done:

Let's use the classic Liederman contraction for an example, start off as shown in the picture (press) the hands together pause for 1-2 seconds, release the pressure for 1second and continue for 40 mini-contractions).

After the mini contractions, hold for a count of 20 seconds. As stated before, the first set will be easy —very easy to be honest.

However, the key is that you are creating cumulative fatigue in the targeted muscle, and the first few reps are fatiguing the slow-twitch fibers, due to the volume of blood, lactic acid buildup and hormonal release that takes place.

THE ISOMETRIC POWER PULSE X40 PROGRAM

17 POWER PULSE X40

By the second set you will be feeling it more than ever. Endurance slow-twitch fibers are starting to burnout, then the fast-twitch endurance fibers begin firing rapidly, and by the 40th rep you will have trouble completing those last few reps due to the intense muscle burn. This really push those endurance fast-twitch fibers for optimum fat-burning and enhanced growth. Isometric pulses works because it targets the motor units hard, coaxing them to rapidly fire mini reps that increases blood volume, lactic acid buildup and hormonal fat-burning properties.

This hits multiple fiber types, and increases tension over-load due to the mini-pulses which will fatigue the endurance fast and slow-twitch fibers, creating intense muscle fiber activation on the muscles involved. While waking up the dormant fibers to fire rapidly. Power Pulses coax more muscle stimulation to more muscle fibers than "traditional" high tension isometric low second contractions. This Program of isometric contraction will lead to a greater degree of lean muscular development.

In other words, moderate tension coupled with extended load time will coax more muscle-building-effects. This activates the target muscle significantly greater and enhances endurance-oriented-fast-twitch muscle fibers to promote muscular growth and strength rapidly.

THE ISOMETRIC POWER PULSE X40 PROGRAM

17 POWER PULSE X40

The primary mechanisms for muscle growth and how they correlate to Isometric Power Pulses are:

1)Continuous tension which increases metabolic stress with contraction type exercises, this blocks blood flow, due to the nature of the exercise and the element of tension being on the muscle's trigger spot.

2)Some exercises increase the muscle's length and resistance is maintained throughout the muscle. This increases various hormonal production which coax the fat-burning effects.

Performing Isometric Power Pulses stimulate the primary mechanics for increasing muscle and fat burning stimulation. By increasing time under load this pre-fatigue the slow-twitch fibers, which enhances an extraordinary amount of endurance fast twitch fibers to fire rapidly. The Isometric Power Pulse x40 Program is a great multi-fat-burning system. That not only burn bodyfat, but increases lean musculature threefold.

The routine hammers away at your muscles within minutes by alternating various muscle groups which receive an accelerated recovery boast because the other muscles are resting or being stretched.

When an isometric curl is performed, your tricep go into an elongated state every time the biceps contract and the same for the triceps. This actually helps the muscles recharge it's batteries for upcoming Isometric sets for great force output.

THE ISOMETRIC POWER PULSE X40 PROGRAM

17 POWER PULSE X40

The Isometric Power Pulse x40 Program is a extra fiber activating enhancer. You will experience that longer tension times coax more growth fibers to fire on extended power contraction reps that follow.
The program builds successful muscle growth due to tension overload with this high rep load technique, you accomplish a lot of workload within a short time frame.

In other words, you will be training each bodypart more frequently through out the week for a more massively hard as nails ripped physique. This brings us to The Isometric Power Pulse X40 muscle-building Program.

THE ISOMETRIC POWER PULSE X40 PROGRAM

17 POWER PULSE X40

HOW TO PERFORM THIS ROUTINE:
THE ISOMETRIC POWER PULSE X40 PROGRAM

Perform the **ISOMETRIC POWER PULSE X40 WORKOUT**—at the contracted position performing 40 mini-contractions (**NON-STOP**). After the mini contractions, hold for a count of 20 seconds. Perform all exercises without rest for 2 rounds.

Alternate day one and day two for 6 days per week for 2 weeks
DAY ONE

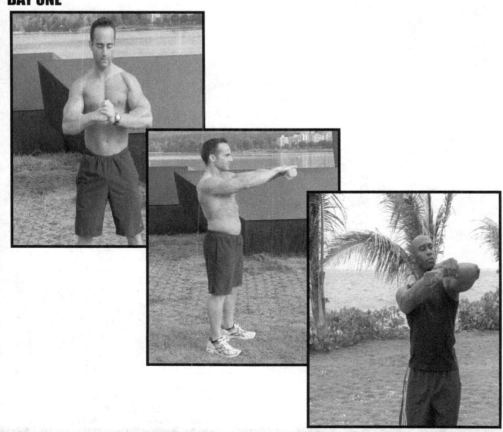

THE ISOMETRIC POWER PULSE X40 PROGRAM

17 POWER PULSE X40

HOW TO PERFORM THIS ROUTINE:
THE ISOMETRIC POWER PULSE X40 PROGRAM

Perform the **ISOMETRIC POWER PULSE X40 WORKOUT**—at the contracted position performing 40 mini-contractions (**NON-STOP**). After the mini contractions, hold for a count of 20 seconds. Perform all exercises without rest for 2 rounds.

DAY ONE continued..........

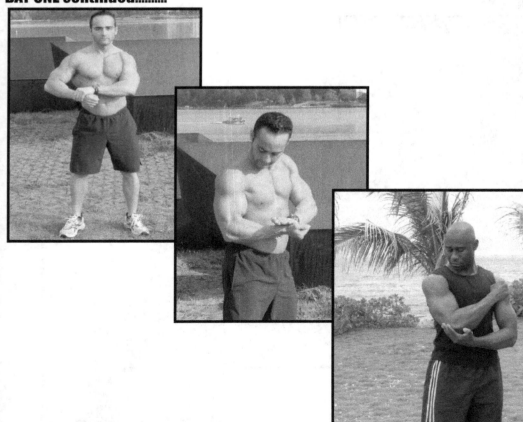

THE ISOMETRIC POWER PULSE X40 PROGRAM

17 POWER PULSE X40

HOW TO PERFORM THIS ROUTINE:
THE ISOMETRIC POWER PULSE X40 PROGRAM

Perform the **ISOMETRIC POWER PULSE X40 WORKOUT**—at the contracted position performing 40 mini-contractions (**NON-STOP**). After the mini contractions, hold for a count of 20 seconds. Perform all exercises without rest for 2 rounds.

DAY ONE continued..........

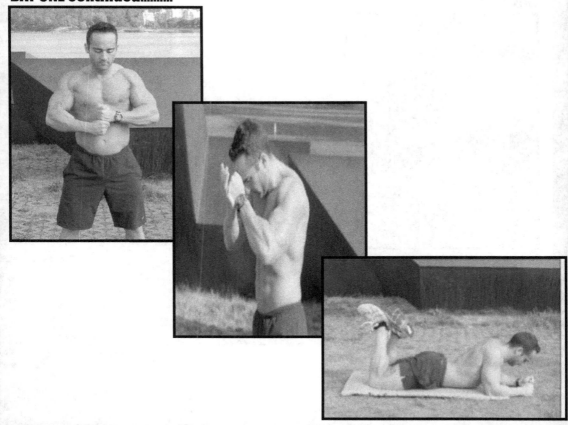

THE ISOMETRIC POWER PULSE X40 PROGRAM

17 POWER PULSE X40

HOW TO PERFORM THIS ROUTINE:
THE ISOMETRIC POWER PULSE X40 PROGRAM

Perform the **ISOMETRIC POWER PULSE X40 WORKOUT**—at the contracted position performing 40 mini-contractions (**NON-STOP**). After the mini contractions, hold for a count of 20 seconds. Perform all exercises without rest for 2 rounds.

DAY TWO

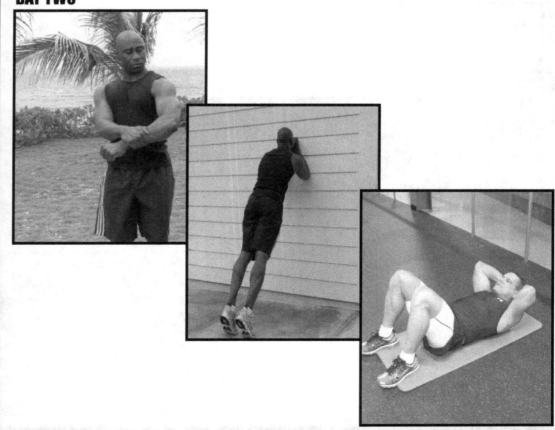

THE ISOMETRIC POWER PULSE X40 PROGRAM

17 POWER PULSE X40

HOW TO PERFORM THIS ROUTINE:
THE ISOMETRIC POWER PULSE X40 PROGRAM

Perform the **ISOMETRIC POWER PULSE X40 WORKOUT**—at the contracted position performing 40 mini-contractions (**NON-STOP**). After the mini contractions, hold for a count of 20 seconds. Perform all exercises without rest for 2 rounds.

DAY TWO continued...........

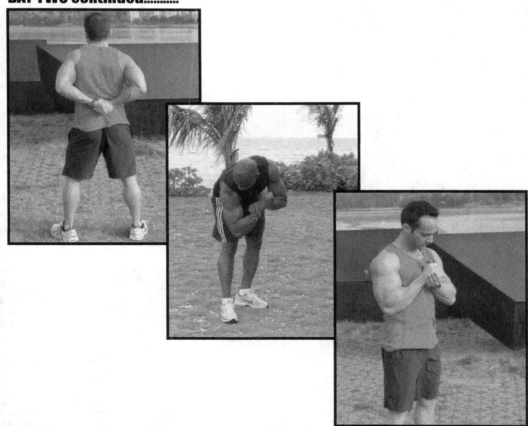

THE ISOMETRIC POWER PULSE PROGRAM

17 POWER PULSE X40

HOW TO PERFORM THIS ROUTINE:
THE ISOMETRIC POWER PULSE X40 PROGRAM

Perform the **ISOMETRIC POWER PULSE X40 WORKOUT**—at the contracted position performing 40 mini-contractions (**NON-STOP**). After the mini contractions, hold for a count of 20 seconds. Perform all exercises without rest for 2 rounds.

DAY TWO continued...........

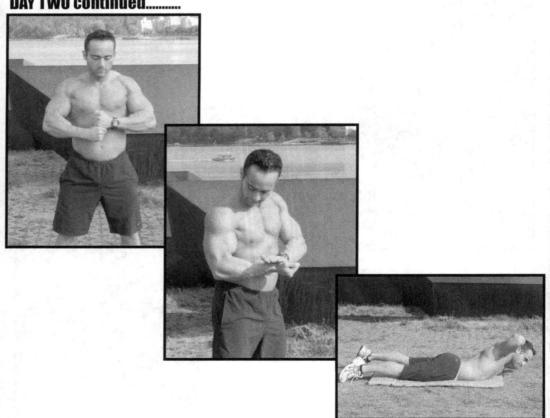

We are looking forward to hearing from you on your progress.
Please drop us an email skippymarl@icloud. com

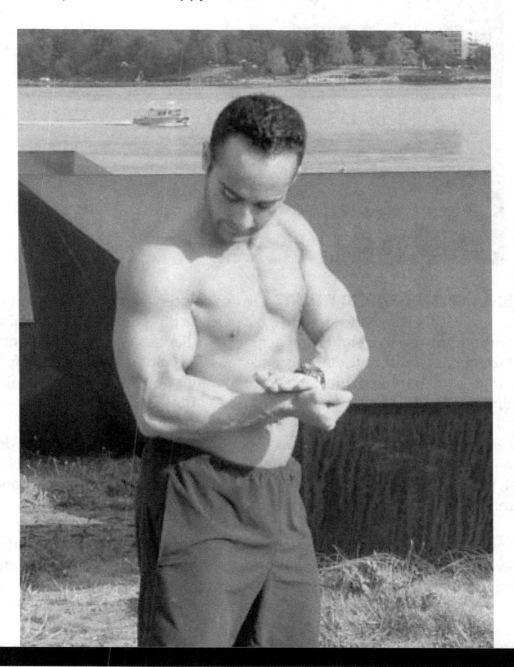

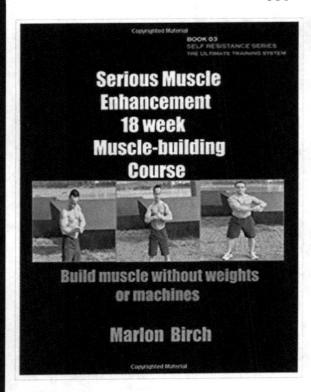

Serious Muscle Enhancement 18 week Muscle-building Course

Build muscle without weights or machines

Marlon Birch

Pack on pounds of muscle fast!

BUILD MUSCLES WITHOUT WEIGHTS Self Resistance when done correctly, will sculpt, reshape and add strength to a person's physique beyond imagination without the use of weights or machines. The Serious Muscle Enhancement Program is the official Self-Resistance muscle-sculpting manual with full-range body-part workouts for every major muscle, with plenty of training tips and tricks to get you building muscles fast.

Learn how to get maximum muscle fiber recruitment and full-muscle development without weights for every body part at every workout. There's a full look at my 18-pound-of-muscle-in-12-weeks original program, and the changes I made to improve the stress methods and results.

You get an innovative muscle-sculpting and strength workout plan without ever having to go to a gym or lift weights. This manual is an absolute must for your muscle-building library, and it's the cornerstone from which most of my programs were created that will take your physique into the fourth dimension!

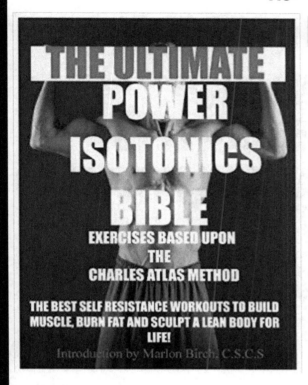

Powerful routines to get in shape!

THE ULTIMATE POWER ISOTONICS BIBLE THE BEST SELF RESISTANCE WORK-OUTS TO BUILD MUSCLE,BURN FAT AND SCULPT A LEAN BODY FOR LIFE!

Do it anywhere, any time, it is the perfect exercise plan all without weights and machines. Build the body of your dreams today. The unique muscle-building exercises in this book will get you growing like crazy because they push your muscles with muscle-building-enhancing exercises and routines with–60 to 90 seconds of tension, which muscles need to increase strength and size.

In this easy-to-read book, you will see illustrations that explain each pro gram—and you will finally see why almost everyone is doing self resistance wrong and why their growth is so painfully slow—Marlon Birch knows the "secrets" on getting amazing muscle size and strength in record time.

He is the ONLY self resistance trainer to take the original Charles Atlas type exercises, enhance them in Hy-brid fashion and became the first ever Professional Bodybuilder using only these exercises to accomplish that goal. Learn from the world's respected fitness trainer and 3-time natural pro body builder be your personal trainer today.

COMING SOON
20TH DECEMBER 2020
TRANSFORMATION CONTEST!

Make a purchase of any of these books save your recite to get a chance to win $$$$$. Contact skippymarl@icloud.com email title (**CONTEST**) Announcements on the way stay tuned.

CPSIA information can be obtained
at www.ICGtesting.com
Printed in the USA
BVHW011016171022
649615BV00008B/169